THE
BEGINNING
RUNNER'S
HANDBOOK

IAN MACNEILL AND
THE SPORT MEDICINE COUNCIL
OF BRITISH COLUMBIA

....

Revised text by
Alison Cristall and Lynda Cannell

THE BEGINNING
RUNNER'S HANDBOOK

|||||||||||||||||||||||||||||||||||||||||||||||||||||||||||||||||||||||||||||||||||||||||

THE PROVEN 13-WEEK RUNWALK PROGRAM

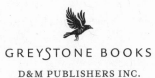

GREYSTONE BOOKS

D&M PUBLISHERS INC.

Vancouver/Toronto/Berkeley

Greystone Books
An imprint of D&M Publishers Inc.
2323 Quebec Street, Suite 201
Vancouver BC Canada V5T 4S7
www.greystonebooks.com

Cataloguing data available from Library and Archives Canada
ISBN 978-1-55365-860-3 (pbk.)
ISBN 978-1-55365-967-9 (ebook)

Edited by Daphne Gray-Grant (original) and Lucy Kenward (fourth edition)
Fourth edition copyedited by Lara Kordic
Cover and text design by Jessica Sullivan
Cover photograph by Jordan Siemens/Getty Images
Illustrations by Warren Clark
Packaged for Greystone Books by House of Words
Printed and bound in Canada by Friesens
Text printed on acid-free, 100% post-consumer paper
Distributed in the U.S. by Publishers Group West

We gratefully acknowledge the financial support of the
Canada Council for the Arts, the British Columbia Arts Council,
the Province of British Columbia through the Book Publishing
Tax Credit and the Government of Canada through the Canada
Book Fund for our publishing activities.

Contents

....

Foreword

....

IT IS IMPOSSIBLE to drive down any road or walk in a park without being reminded that many people choose running as a way to maintain or improve their health. Running has gained popularity not only because it requires scant equipment and is portable to any site, but also because it has been proven to reduce the risk of such conditions as heart disease, high blood pressure, diabetes, obesity and depression. Regular exercise is known to extend people's years of active and independent living. And to get these benefits requires an outlay of just a few hours each week. Small wonder that hundreds of thousands of enthusiasts around the world find running an ideal form of exercise and a good path to physical fitness.

This book is aimed at the would-be runner who needs information about how to become fit. Running appears to be so simple that many individuals approach it thinking success will come easily; beginning runners often get hurt because they train too intensely and too frequently. Simply put, many individuals mistakenly assume that more exercise is better, but an overdose of running can invite injury. The moderate, 13-week RunWalk program and the guidance offered in this book equip an aspiring runner with the knowledge essential to achieving his or her goal—whether that be running for long-term fitness or preparing to participate in a 10-k event—in manageable stages, with minimal risk of injury.

As a former Olympic runner, and coach to dozens of Olympic runners over the past 55 years, I believe in the intrinsic value of running. But as a sport medicine specialist, I know that most of the more than half-million patients entering the clinic with which I am associated have been runners. Had they followed a program like the one presented here, it is far less likely that they would have had to seek medical treatment. This book offers the most concise presentation of information for the beginning runner I have ever seen. I recommend it to every reader as the path to a healthy fitness routine and a more enjoyable life.

DOUG CLEMENT, M.D.

Introduction

....

THIS BOOK was written specifically for *beginning* runners. It has been designed to answer the practical questions you may have about getting started. It will tell you how to avoid sore muscles and injury. It will give you advice about motivation and help you set realistic and achievable goals. And, most important, it will provide you with a recipe for success, a tried-and-true training program for starting to run.

The heart and soul of this book is SportMedBC's 13-week program that has its roots in what is now one of the world's most popular 10-k events, the *Vancouver Sun* Run™. A relatively obscure event when it started in 1983, the *Vancouver Sun* Run™ annually attracts 50,000+ runners and walkers. As the run started to grow, event organizers noticed that the frequency of running-related injuries had risen. A good number of the runners were first-timers, and many of them hadn't properly trained or prepared for the event. It wasn't until after they were injured that they learned the necessary steps required to safely go the distance. Either that, or they quit altogether.

It seemed clear that many participants would benefit from receiving expert advice *before* the event.

The 13-week training program presented in this book was originally conceived by Dr. Doug Clement, a sport medicine physician, former Canadian national team running coach and retired co-director of the Allan McGavin Sport Medicine Centre at the University of British Columbia. After several years of treating a steady stream of running casualties, he decided to design a training plan that neophyte runners could follow and benefit from. The mandate was simple: develop a graduated program that intersperses walking with jogging or running in order to help people develop the physical robustness to run, walk or jog a 10-k course without getting injured.

In 1996, the 13-week RunWalk program became the basis for a series of community-based running clinics created and managed by SportMedBC. Clinics are available at local recreation centers, fitness clubs and YMCAS/YWCAS. Although the fundamentals of the program stayed the same (walking interspersed with jogging or running), each training segment was carefully fine-tuned. Over five years, the original training program was then modified to fit the real-life experiences of the more than 75,000 individuals who had used the program. Compelled by the testimonials of clinic participants—some of whom claimed that following the program provided one of the most rewarding, life-altering experiences they had ever had—we decided to take the program to a larger audience. Since then, tens of thousands of people worldwide have accomplished their running goals using the *Beginning Runner's Handbook*.

This program has been proven to work by people who may have been fearful at first, but who doggedly set goals and persevered to achieve them. The book includes first-hand accounts from many of these runners—telling about their challenges, setbacks, successes and failures. As well, it includes guidance from a wide range of professionals, all experts in their respective fields of nutrition, sport medicine, sport science, psychology and coaching, and running tips from track-and-field Olympian and RunWalk coach Lynn Kanuka.

Whether you want to start running to lose weight, relieve stress, quit smoking, reduce your cholesterol levels, meet new people or simply get fitter, this book will help you meet your goal. You will learn how to start an exercise regime the right way, and you will be able to learn from the mistakes and successes of others. Best of all, once you have started the program, you will be able to come back to the book and review specific sections for encouragement, advice and reinforcement. Having the book is a bit like having a personal running coach in your back pocket. If you use a logbook, and we highly recommend that you do, this book will also help serve as a permanent record of your achievement. (See Resources and References, page 207, for information on SportMedBC's 13-week training log, which is designed specifically to accompany the program.)

A word of caution. As you thumb through the book and flip to the training program itself, you may at first glance think the 13-week RunWalk program looks too easy. You may wonder what walking has to do with training to become a runner. The answer is that your bones, ligaments, tendons and muscles require a very slow and gradual buildup to activity, particularly if they haven't seen much action for a while; walking helps prepare them for the stress of running. Although you may be tempted to go out and just start running on your own, or to jump ahead, you should stick to the program. There is no magic potion you can swallow to become a runner, no shortcuts or untold secrets of success. The 13-week program requires dedication and a certain amount of perseverance.

We do know, however, that it works. Even if you have no intention of toeing up to the start line of a race, consider making a commitment to follow the program. At the end of the 13 weeks, you will feel better and you'll be healthier as well. Who knows? You might even become a runner for life.

1

Why Run?

....

ONLY A few decades ago, running was considered the sport of odd-balls and kooks; few recognized its health benefits. Although today it is widely accepted that fit people are healthier and live longer, it took some rigorous research to prove the point.

One of the first persons to shed light on the exercise/health debate was British researcher J.N. Morris. In the 1960s, he studied the illness rates of conductors and drivers working the London buses, and of mail carriers and their deskbound counterparts inside post offices. He discovered that the conductors and mail carriers, who were constantly moving, suffered fewer heart attacks than did the more sedentary drivers and clerks. Furthermore, when the conductors and carriers did have heart attacks, they usually survived, whereas the drivers and clerks more often died.

American researcher Ralph Paffenbarger conducted a similar study in 1968, comparing the health of longshoremen with that of dockside office workers. His findings mirrored those of Morris: the fitter the workers were, the longer they lived. That still left an important question: why? To appreciate the answer, you need to understand a little bit about how the human body operates.

THE IMPORTANCE OF OXYGEN

Every living cell in the body requires a constant supply of oxygen. Oxygen is absorbed into the blood via the lungs, then transported throughout the body by means of a system of blood vessels, the largest of which are the veins and arteries, the smallest the capillaries. In addition to inherited health factors, both fitness and diet affect how efficiently a person's oxygen delivery system functions.

Unfortunately, not only are people in the Western world sedentary, they also often have diets high in saturated fat. That fat gets into the bloodstream and lodges in cracks in the arterial walls in a form called plaque. Over time the plaque builds, so that eventually it can block the flow of oxygenated blood to major organs such as the heart and brain as well as to the muscles. If the heart receives too little oxygen, the result can be angina. With angina, which can be very painful, the heart seizes momentarily but recovers its momentum when the supply of oxygen kicks in again. But if the flow of oxygen is cut off for long enough, the result will be a myocardial infarction, or as it's more commonly known, a heart attack.

Another consequence of poor circulation can be a blockage of blood to the brain, leading to a stroke. With a mild stroke, parts of an oxygen-deprived brain simply die off, often resulting in paralysis or the loss of certain functions. A more extensive stroke can be fatal.

Our muscles also need oxygen for almost everything they do. Generally, the harder they work, the more oxygen they need. But sudden surges of energy, such as that needed by someone fleeing from a grizzly bear, for example, require hardly any oxygen at all. That's because the body has more than one way of producing energy.

The aerobic and anaerobic systems

The word "aerobic" means "in the presence of oxygen." You are operating aerobically when you walk, sit, sleep, eat, watch television or read a book and, ideally, when you exercise

FACT

Running two to three times a week can reduce your risk of gallstone disease by 20 to 40 percent, according to a 1997 study by the Harvard School of Public Health at Harvard Medical School.

FACT

A 1997 study at Harvard University found that women who exercise produce a less potent form of estrogen than those who do not. The study concluded that women who exercise can halve their risk of developing breast and uterine cancer.

("ideally" because when your body operates aerobically, it can produce energy to keep you going for a long time). In the simplest terms, you produce energy aerobically when the air you breathe works together with the food you eat to make your muscles operate. It's similar to the way gas and air work together to make a car's engine go.

Sometimes your body is called upon to do strenuous work very quickly—for example, to help you flee when you suddenly find yourself between a bear and her cubs. To have any chance of escaping, you will have to come up with a lot of energy almost instantly. That's when your anaerobic system is likely to kick in. As the name suggests, anaerobic means "in the absence of oxygen." Unlike the aerobic system, which requires oxygen to produce energy, the anaerobic system uses the fuel stored in the muscles.

Day to day, your body gets its energy from a mix of aerobic and anaerobic sources. The more intense the activity and the more your body's demand for oxygen exceeds your ability to supply it, the more you work anaerobically. That's why when you're engaged in intense activity, your breathing accelerates: your body is trying to get more of that precious oxygen and remain aerobic.

RUNNER PROFILE

Jack

JACK took up running more than 35 years ago. At the time, he had his heart set on a career as a professional football player, and running seemed like a great way to improve his endurance. He participated in the first Vancouver Marathon in 1972, one of only 32 brave enough, or perhaps, some would have said at the time, foolish enough to do so. Eventually his gridiron dreams receded, but his love of running remained. A sport medicine physician and co-director of a large university sport medicine center, Jack's not sure how he'd get through a week without running. Currently in his 60s, he has run more than 60 marathons and is still going strong.

Everyone, even a highly trained athlete, works anaerobically in certain situations. A wide receiver going for a pass in a football game, for example, will produce energy anaerobically when he or she is sprinting down the sideline in pursuit of the ball. As you become fitter, however, you will push up your "anaerobic threshold," the point at which your body switches over to anaerobic-based energy sources.

The reason you want to push up your anaerobic threshold is that if you are getting your energy from mainly anaerobic sources, you can't keep up any activity for very long. Depending on how fit you are, your anaerobic energy supply will last from 5 to 60 seconds. Obviously that's not enough to allow you to run around the block, let alone run 10 k.

Another reason to prolong the amount of time you work aerobically is that the chemical reactions taking place in your body during anaerobic exercise produce accumulations of lactic acid in the working muscles. Researchers think this byproduct is the cause of the soreness in muscles following bouts of strenuous exercise. Again, depending on how fit you are, your body will take a day or more to break down and eliminate the lactic acid.

Feeling a little stiff and sore after a workout isn't entirely bad; it's part of the process that will make you fitter. Still, the 13-week RunWalk program will slowly increase your tolerance for exercise while keeping your body working aerobically as much as possible. As you gradually train yourself, you will find you are able to function more efficiently (that is, aerobically) at higher workloads.

EXERCISE AND HEALTH

How does being fit make you healthier?

The blood vessels of a fit person tend to accumulate less plaque than those of an unfit person, leading to a lower risk of heart attack or stroke. Additionally, a person who exercises will improve his or her circulatory system in general, in part by making the lining of the blood vessels more flexible, so that the heart doesn't have to work as hard to pump the blood through the body. The result is that even if there are blockages in the blood vessels, the circulation around those blockages will improve. (There's still some debate about whether you can actually reduce the amount of plaque that's already built up in your system, but the question might be moot if you can improve the circulation around it.)

Over time, as you exercise regularly you increase the number of capillaries in your muscles (the small blood vessels that deliver nutrients and remove wastes), as well as the number of mitochondria (living particles inside cells that produce energy) and the enzymes in those mitochondria that allow you to function aerobically.

Exercise stimulates the body to produce endorphins, the body's natural painkillers. Endorphins are remarkably similar in structure to morphine, and there's some evidence that people get addicted to running because they are hooked on the endorphin rush. There are less healthy things to be hooked on!

Moderate exercise also seems to boost the immune system, apparently by improving the killer T-cell function. These cells are the army ants of your immune system; they rush in and

RUNNER PROFILE

Holly

AS A TEACHER and mother of two, Holly never felt like she had time to exercise. Before having kids she was an avid runner, but over the past four years she seemed to be consumed with family and work, never leaving time for herself. Realizing she needed to make a change, Holly signed up for a 13-week RunWalk clinic. At first she was fearful she would not be able to run three times a week, but after negotiating babysitting duties with her husband, she was soon running once the kids went to bed. "It was so important to feel like me again. It's so easy to make excuses and not exercise; nothing beats going for a run to re-energize me. I think it even makes me a better mom."

kill invaders. (But note that if you exercise until your body is thoroughly fatigued, you can actually impair killer T-cell function. During the 24 to 48 hours following exhaustive exercise—a marathon, for example—you are more susceptible to upper respiratory system infections, such as colds.)

Finally, exercise reduces stress. It does this by allowing the body to metabolize the stress hormone adrenaline more quickly. Adrenaline is one of nature's mixed blessings, vital to get you through crises but debilitating if there's too much of it or if it sticks around too long. Better regulation of the amount of adrenaline in your system is another potential health benefit of exercise.

MORE REASONS TO GET FIT

Regular exercise provides a great incentive for adopting a healthier lifestyle—eating a low-fat diet, getting proper rest, forgoing cigarettes—because doing so makes exercise easier and more pleasant.

Exercise can help you control your weight. Many people put on weight as they age. Some argue it's because the metabolism slows with age; others say the only reason the metabolism slows down is that people become less active as they get older. (Then again, some people remain slim their entire lives and never seem to do a stitch of work.) What is known for certain is that most people find a regular exercise program—combined with healthy eating habits—can help ward off extra pounds. And speaking of exercise and food, there's a little bonus built into life for people who exercise. Even if weight is not an issue for you, doing more exercise (that is, burning more calories) opens up room in your diet for more of the things you love to eat that would otherwise add inches to your waistline, hips or buttocks.

Fit people have a better self-image, partly because they look and feel better and partly because they have more confidence in their ability to be active. Perhaps this is the basis for the belief that fit people make better lovers!

FACT

Running lowers your blood pressure and your resting heart rate while raising your "good" cholesterol levels.

In any case, getting fit will make you stronger, so you can enjoy participating in a broader range of physical activities. If you're the kind of person who cringes in fear when one of the kids suggests going to the park and kicking a ball around, getting in shape can improve not only your life but your children's as well. Active parents encourage a more active lifestyle in their children, not just when the kids are young but in all the years to come.

Staying active as you age is the most powerful tool to living a long and healthy life. Endurance activities such as running have proven anti-aging effects on the brain, skin, hair, gonads (ovaries and testicles), kidneys, spleen and liver. Exercise has benefits for people even when they start after age 65.

THE JOY OF RUNNING

Aerobic exercise increases the heart rate and thereby helps to improve your cardiovascular system, stave off heart disease and improve circulation and muscle tone. It can provide you with more energy, perhaps help you lose weight, probably make you sleep better and certainly make you look and feel a lot better about yourself. But of all the possible forms of aerobic activity, why choose running?

For starters, running is one of the least expensive sports. Once you invest in a good pair of shoes, you're done. Compare this with the cost of golf, skiing, hockey or even tennis. With running, there are no green fees to pay, lift tickets to buy, pads to wear through or balls to wear out.

Running is also easy to get involved in. All it takes is a pair of good shoes, a little time and a healthy dose of motivation. You can do it practically anywhere. Some people like to run alongside busy streets, others on tree-shaded park trails. Some like to jog along the beach at sunset; some run in the dead of night among deserted skyscrapers. You can run alone just as easily as in the middle of a pack. You can go the competitive route and enter races, or spend the rest of your life in pursuit

Excessive pooling of blood in the legs because of inactivity may cause varicose veins. Exercise can help provide an efficient return of venous blood to the heart after it has been pumped to other parts of your body.

of personal goals, never bothering to check your time and distance, simply running for the sheer joy and benefits of it.

You can run your whole life. With proper conditioning, your body will run well into old age.

Running is something you can do with friends or alone. You don't need other people the way you do with tennis, racquetball, soccer, hockey, basketball or Frisbee. You don't have to wait for someone to meet you, then feel stuck when the person doesn't show up. You can warm up, run for 20 minutes, cool down, shower and get on with the rest of your day, just like that.

If you do choose to run by yourself, running can give you something you may have difficulty finding in your life: time to get away from it all and be alone with your own thoughts.

People who are physically fit usually have lower resting heart rates and blood pressure levels. They are less susceptible to the effects of stress, which causes heart rate and blood pressure to rise.

WHEN Paul was approaching 50, his life took a downturn. "I developed rheumatoid arthritis and all of a sudden I had a nervous breakdown," the now 56-year-old salesman says.

Deeply concerned for his health and well-being, both his doctor and his psychiatrist recommended more exercise. Paul joined a walking club, which not only got him moving but helped break down the emotional barriers he'd built up around himself. Finding himself at the front of the walking pack eventually gave him the confidence to start running, and soon afterward the dividends of exercise and a healthier lifestyle started rolling in. "Running helped me get a grip on my arthritis and gave me the energy to recover from my depression. It also helped me stop distancing myself from other people."

Today, Paul thinks of running as the thread that helps tie his life together. "The bad things that happened to me were kind of a wake-up call. I'd still like to lose some weight and run a little faster," he says with a chuckle, "but at least I haven't put on any more weight and I'm running faster now than if I'd never started."

RUNNER PROFILE

Paul

If you have a busy career and/or a growing family, you can sometimes feel pretty squeezed. Everybody needs some time alone, and running can give you that time.

Alternatively, running can help you make new friends. If you choose to join a running group, you will meet people you might never have met in other circumstances—people whose other interests in life are entirely different from yours. Doctors run with dockworkers who run with flight attendants who run with writers who run with factory workers, and so on. People who run together accept each other as equals.

Running can teach you a lot about who you are. It can show you your limitations and give you the opportunity to move past them. If you keep raising the bar, running can give you the tremendous feeling that bars were made to be raised. Running takes commitment, determination, desire, hard work and a sense of self-worth. Think how many other areas in your life could benefit from your having these attributes.

CHAPTER 1 SUMMARY

1. The 13-week RunWalk program will slowly increase your tolerance for exercise. As you gradually train yourself, you will be able to function aerobically at higher workloads.
2. Exercise will help lower the risk of heart attack or stroke, boost your immune system and reduce stress.
3. Being physically fit will help control your weight. Ultimately, people who exercise are shown to have a better self-image.
4. Running is a great way to stay fit. All you need is a pair of running shoes.
5. You can choose to run by yourself or join a group. Although it takes commitment and desire to stick with a running program, in the end the commitment will help you in all aspects of your life.

2

Getting Ready to Run

....

MOST PEOPLE can lace up their shoes and start a running program without worrying about bringing on a heart attack, aggravating a bad back or provoking some other medical catastrophe. A small percentage, however, should consult a doctor before starting any fitness regimen, whether or not it includes running.

One way to decide if you need medical supervision is to take a physical readiness test. The Canadian Society for Exercise Physiology has developed a good one, called the Physical Activity Readiness Questionnaire, or PAR-Q, for short (page 30). If you get through the questionnaire without answering yes to any of the questions—and it's in your best interest to answer them honestly—then you can probably start an exercise program without fear of hurting yourself.

If, however, you answer yes to one or more of these questions, you should talk to your doctor before proceeding.

If you want to get a more accurate assessment of your physical condition, ask your doctor to do a Physical Activity Readiness Medical Examination (the PARmed-X, for short) with you. This special checklist includes useful advice on what types of exercises persons with certain underlying physical conditions can do safely. There's even a special screening tool for pregnant women considering an exercise program. Pregnancy rarely makes exercise inadvisable, but it's wise to check with a qualified professional.

THE THREE RULES OF EXERCISE

Once you're cleared to start an exercise program, it's time to memorize the three rules of exercise: moderation, consistency and rest. They're simple rules, and if you live by them you will find that moving from a sedentary life to an active one can be quite enjoyable rather than a trip through training hell. You will also go a long way toward avoiding injuries, which can undo months, even years, of work.

Of course, living by the three rules will not make you invulnerable to pain or injury. But these rules will help ease you to a higher level of fitness by subjecting your body to the proper amount of stress.

Rule 1: Be moderate

Start slowly. Even if you already have a good level of cardio-vascular fitness from other sports, you should follow this advice. Being able to cycle in the Tour de France or swim the English Channel doesn't make you a runner. Even experienced runners (and walkers) need to take care not to overstress themselves. That's because there are special musculoskeletal stresses peculiar to running.

The cardiovascular system is considerably more robust than the musculoskeletal system. Given a reasonable amount of stress, it will respond eagerly, quickly strengthening and giving you the ability to transport more oxygen to hungry muscles. Unfortunately, your bones, ligaments, tendons and muscles are not quite as adaptable. According to Dr. Tim Noakes, an exercise science and sport medicine research director at the University of Cape Town and co-author of *Running Injuries*, "If you're reasonably athletic, after six months or so of training you could technically run in a marathon, but your bones wouldn't be up to it yet." He says the majority of people who haven't been very active are susceptible to bone stress fractures in the first three to six months if they continually push their training. In other words, while your heart and lungs may be urging you to go, your bones, ligaments, tendons and muscles may want you to ease up.

A large number of well-intentioned people derail their fitness programs by being immoderate. Many of them make a New Year's resolution to get in shape and crowd the fitness centers during the first couple of weeks of January, but drop out by the time spring rolls around. Those who aren't injured grow discouraged by the punishing pace to which they've subjected themselves.

Although the human body can withstand a great deal of stress, to avoid injury you must apply this stress gradually. That's why we advise you to not jump ahead in the training program described in this book, even if it seems somewhat "lightweight" to you in the beginning. Skipping ahead will not make you fit faster, but it will significantly increase the risk that you will be sidelined with sore muscles and joints, or worse.

Rule 2: Be consistent

If moderation is the first rule of training, consistency is the second. Those who break Rule 1 invariably break Rule 2. Here's the pattern. You decide to get in shape, so you head to the gym or go for as long a run as you can endure, and for the next week you feel as though you've been run over by a truck. By the time you've recovered enough to take another stab at it, you push yourself to the wall again to make up for lost time. This kind of training isn't training at all. It's doing you more harm than good, and because it makes you feel worse rather than better, soon common sense kicks in and undermines your commitment. Eventually you quit.

The virtues of consistency cannot be overstated. When you work out consistently, your body has more time to adapt to the stress of training. What's more, if you are consistent, you won't have to make up for lost time. A day or two of extra-hard work will not make up for those missed training sessions. Instead, you are more likely to overstress your body and find yourself back at square one—or, worse, facing an illness or injury.

As well, the longer you spend developing a solid fitness base, the more secure it is, which means you can take a break every now and then without blowing your whole game plan.

If you think carefully about Rules 1 and 2, it's easy to see why fit people make training part of their lives. The idea that training never ends may seem daunting in the beginning, especially if you find your first efforts difficult. But once your body and mind begin to benefit from exercise, you will find yourself craving it. Instead of forcing yourself to do it, you'll be worrying about when you are going to get the chance. Fit people typically reach stages in their day or week when they are champing at the bit to tie on their shoes and go.

RUNNER PROFILE

Marcel

MARCEL had his first heart attack when he was just 57. "I guess if you want to look on the bright side," he says, "it was something of a wake-up call." An avid tennis player, Marcel figured he'd be taking it pretty easy for the rest of his life after he collapsed in the shower following a particularly tough tennis match. "I always knew exercise was the way to prevent heart disease, but I figured once you went down you had to sort of back off."

His doctor disagreed and encouraged him to change his lifestyle and stop exercising in fits and starts. "He told me I could do a lot more exercise than I was used to; it was a matter of building up to it slowly and doing a few other things differently in my life." He was referred to a nutritionist, who overhauled his diet, and six months after his heart attack Marcel was much healthier, running three times a week and playing a stronger tennis game than ever.

Rule 3: Give your body time to rest

Rest gives your body time and energy to adapt to the changes you bring to it by training. Once your body has adapted, you'll be stronger and more efficient. Build time for rest and recovery into your training plan and be sure to space your workouts over the entire week, not pile them up in a few days.

Think of rest the same way you think of your training sessions—as a conscious physical activity essential to your program and your well-being. Rest is not the avoidance of work; it is a proper period of recovery from an activity that wears your body down.

WHERE TO RUN

One of the great things about running is that you can do it practically anywhere—on a road, in a park, around a track, across the country or on the spot. Nonetheless, if you have a choice, running on softer surfaces will reduce the stress and strain on bones, ligaments, tendons and muscles and make your run more enjoyable all around.

As a running surface, asphalt is preferable to concrete and dirt is better yet because it will absorb more of the impact. If concrete, which does not absorb any impact, is the worst surface, grass or rubberized tracks are probably the best, mainly because they absorb the most. Some runners find tracks boring. However, grass can hide holes or tree roots that can make you trip. Consider your options carefully.

TRAIL RUNNING

Trail running is quickly becoming the fastest-growing segment of running. Trails can range from level paths to hundreds of feet of elevation gain and loss. The benefits of running on softer surfaces in natural terrain range from the physiological to the psychological. Physically, trails provide a much more forgiving surface that decreases the impact on joints. Psychologically, trail running can also alleviate any boredom you might have with your regular running routine. It's a great way to get off the pavement, out of the gym and into nature. Keep in mind that your body needs to acclimate to the trails: the softer surface absorbs quite a bit more energy, and initially you'll have to work a little harder.

Tips for trail-running safety

> Don't set out on a long trip without training.
> Don't venture out on your own.
> Know the trail and watch your footing.
> Let people know where you are going to be and how long you expect to be out for.
> Show respect for the weather and weather forecasts; be prepared for bad weather and cold, even on short trips.

THE PROBLEM WITH FEET

Footwear has come a long way in the last 20 years, and today's modern shoes can not only help counter various foot flaws but also absorb a lot of the shock to which running subjects your body.

Barefoot running

Long before running shoes, people ran barefoot in their natural environment. The reclusive Tarahumara natives of Mexico's Copper Canyon, for example, have been running ultramarathon distances in minimal footwear for generations. And while few people compete barefoot, some runners have achieved great success without shoes. Ethiopia's Abebe Bikila won gold in the men's marathon at the 1960 Summer Olympics in Rome, Italy, in a time of two hours and 15 minutes, and in the 1980s South Africa's Zola Budd twice broke the world record in the women's 5,000 meters and was a two-time winner at the World Cross-Country Championships.

Recently, there's been a whole lot more hype about barefoot running. According to Dr. Christopher MacLean, director of biomechanics at the Paris Orthotics Lab Division in Vancouver, the excitement started in the spring of 2009 with the publication of Christopher McDougall's book, *Born to Run,* a book about the running feats of the Tarahumara. In the fall of that same year, a study by Dr. Casey Kerrigan and others. found that the stress load on the knees and hips may be increased when running in running shoes rather than in bare feet. The media therefore concluded that it was healthier to run without running shoes. However, MacLean suggests that the results of this study should be viewed with caution, as "an increase in joint movement may be healthier depending on an individual's alignment."

As more studies take place, some evidence now supports the proposed benefits of running barefoot, including increased proprioception (the ability of the foot and ankle to sense motion and position relative to the rest of the body) and increased strength and activation in these same small muscles.

Pronation and supination

Phil Moore, owner of Vancouver's LadySport, has a tremendous amount of expertise on athletic footwear. He believes that the human foot is remarkably well adapted to the work required of it. "In terms of mechanics, the rear foot and forefoot are working on different planes. As you land on your heel and go into the mid-stance, the foot acts like a loose bag of bones. It does this both to absorb the shock and to adapt to various anomalies in the surface you are running on. When it operates efficiently and properly and there aren't any obtuse angles that shouldn't be there, the foot works really well."

Unfortunately, not all feet work equally well. Moore says that about 95 percent of the problem feet he sees are afflicted by overpronation, which is a tendency for the foot to roll too far inward. (Notice that the problem is *over*pronation. The foot pronates naturally. If it didn't, it would have a tough time absorbing the shock of running.)

The overpronated foot can cause several problems, both in the foot itself and in the rest of the leg, not to mention in the

FACT

Pronation is the flattening of your foot's arch during weight bearing, causing the foot to roll inward. Some pronation is normal and allows your foot to absorb shock. Excessive pronation, however, will strain your foot, knee, leg, thigh and hip.

Supination occurs when
your foot's arch fails to
flatten out enough dur-
ing weight bearing. If
you suffer from excess
supination—a rare con-
dition—you'll tend to
walk on the outside
edges of your feet.

lower back. Before the design of footwear became the science
it is today, overpronated feet were called flat feet, and people
with such feet were often kept out of the army because they
couldn't walk or run long distances. If you stand up and arti-
ficially flatten your feet, you'll notice that your knees start
pointing inward. If you run that way, your knees will track
poorly and joint problems could develop. A flat foot also com-
presses the lower back and can lead to back pain.

The opposite of pronation is supination, which occurs
when the foot's arch fails to flatten out enough during weight
bearing. If you have this rare condition, you'll tend to walk on
the outside edges of your feet.

Some people start out with good feet but life plays havoc
with them. For example, the weight of pregnancy can cause
a woman's feet to flatten, especially if she regularly wears
sandals. Often, people don't notice flaws in their feet when
they are young and flexible, but when those people get older
or put more stress on their feet by running, the flaws become
apparent.

RUNNING SHOE TRENDS

Over the past 10 years, the biggest trend in running shoes has
been a move toward more "neutral" shoes. "Initially, runners thought that adding more stability to their shoes would
be good. In the end, shoes were overcorrecting people," says
Rand Clement, Alliance Athletic partner and owner of The
Right Shoe in Vancouver. "Neutral shoes," he added, "ended
up being supportive enough for most people." More supportive shoes used to wear out quickly, leading to more injuries;
now shoes in general are becoming less structured but more
responsive. As he points out, people wearing orthotics have
had a big influence on the sales of neutral shoes. A corrective
orthotic in a big beefy shoe doesn't make sense. An orthotic
in a neutral shoe allows a runner to have the right amount of
stability without being overcorrected.

Rand Clement is often asked, "Can I wear my trendy athletic 'street' shoes for running?" His response is, "Potentially, but with the move toward minimalist shoes, it's not an easy question to answer anymore. At a minimum, the shoe should be an athletic shoe." Most importantly, the shoe needs to have some function, some cushioning or support. He recommends bringing your shoe into a running store and having the staff take a look at them. "That way a beginning runner can get properly fitted at the store and know whether their trendy athletic 'street' shoes are appropriate or not."

Today many high-level track athletes focus part of their training on barefoot running. They run on a track or a field without harmful debris or other hazards, and they often wear a minimalist shoe that protects their foot but does not provide the cushioning or structure seen in most modern running shoes. Many technical running shoe companies have launched a minimalist shoe, as barefoot running and minimalist shoes are a fad that is not fizzling. So, is barefoot running a good thing?

Like Rand Clement, Dr. MacLean explains, "It is likely that the healthiest way to run is in an appropriately designed running shoe that is best suited for the runner's foot type and biomechanics. Minimalist footwear should only be considered after consulting with a knowledgeable foot care specialist, a running coach and/or a reputable technical running shoe retailer."

"For a beginning runner," says Dr. MacLean, "shoes are not the issue. Running style or form is. For example, there is evidence that increasing your running cadence (how many steps you take per minute) decreases the torque (rotational force) at the hip and knee, perhaps reducing your chance of injury." In general, then, while the shoes are moving off the shelf, minimalist shoes and barefoot running are only appropriate for high-level runners who are free from injury and can train in a safe environment, on a well-maintained track or field. Says

MacLean, "People are buying them, but they need to incorporate the shoes gradually into their training routine. Don't go and throw out your cushioned running shoes! If you really must try the latest fad, start with 10 minutes of running in minimalist shoes and build from there."

Toner shoes are athletic sneakers that feature an extremely pronounced convex-rounded sole. Many companies claim these shoes will improve posture, ease back pain and, lately, help tone your thighs and buttocks. According to many experts, these shoes are not appropriate for running but may be beneficial for some walking programs. The front of the shoe is quite high and the heel is quite low, which mimics the effect of standing on a wobble board or an uneven surface. These shoes cause the muscles in the back of the leg to fire while trying to keep you balanced. If you have problems with your forefoot, these shoes may provide a natural rolling motion so your foot has to flex less. For people without forefoot problems, these shoes will not have any negative effect on the foot's natural flex and will not lead to injury.

CHOOSING A GOOD SHOE
When you run, each foot strikes the ground somewhere between 800 and 1,200 times per mile (500 and 750 times per kilometer). In the beginning, you will be coming down on your feet with one and one-half to two times your body weight, but when you get faster the impact can increase to four times your body weight. For that reason alone your footwear needs increased cushioning throughout, particularly in the heel. It also has to provide good support for the foot and arch. Women should remember that they generally have narrower feet than men and might have trouble fitting securely into men's shoes. Fortunately, shoe manufacturers have recognized this market. Every good running shoe company now offers separate styles for men and women. And some, such as New Balance, also offer shoes in various widths.

You may already have had hints of foot problems. Perhaps you never seem to be able to buy shoes that feel right, or you develop various pains in your feet, legs or lower body if you walk for any length of time. Today there is likely a shoe to help you overcome your problems. The best way to find the right shoe for you is to go to a good running store and have your foot measured properly by a running shoe expert. Once you have this information, you will be better able to choose the correct shoe style for your feet.

Stable shoes that correct or support the alignment of your feet will help you to run efficiently and without pain. If your feet overpronate, you need shoes that provide extra support so that your feet don't flatten out too much. Sometimes there's enough support in the shoes; sometimes you have to add some kind of orthotic (shoe insert), which can be prescribed by a sport physician or podiatrist. When you do find shoes that work for you, you'll probably want to stick with that model as long as it is available because people often develop problems just after switching to another type of shoe.

In choosing shoes, it's also important to think about the type of surface you run on. If you have a normal or "neutral" foot, you still might want a shoe with more support if you run on trails or other uneven ground, where there is more chance of twisting an ankle.

Shoe quality varies considerably; no two pairs are identical. (It's said that cars made on Mondays and Fridays have more defects and the same is probably true when it comes to shoes.) Inspect shoes carefully before buying and ask your retailer about the return policy for defective ones, because defects often show up only after the shoe is put to the test of use. If you're not happy with the retailer's policy, shop somewhere else; most manufacturers of better-quality running shoes offer a warranty on their product. After you take your shoes home, remember to inspect them regularly so that you spot deterioration before it can cause a running injury.

> **TIP**
>
> If you have a
> > "normal" foot, look for a stability shoe with moderate control features and a semi-curved last (inner sole).
> > "flat" foot, try a motion control or stability shoe, with a firm midsole and a straight or semi-curved last.
> > high-arched foot, lace up a neutral cushioned shoe with good flexibility (stay away from motion control shoes) and a curved last.

Walking puts less stress on your feet than running, but walking in the wrong type of shoes will also lead to misery. Your feet support you and carry you for miles, not only when you're walking for exercise but through every step of your life. Comfortable, flexible, lightweight walking shoes, with a cushioned sole, good arch support, a firm heel counter and a little extra room for your toes, are a very worthwhile investment.

CHOOSING YOUR CLOTHING

Clothing is not the most important consideration when you run, but it's not irrelevant either. What you wear should be primarily a function of weather. Stores offer a lot of flashy running gear, but consider comfort first.

PLAGUED by lower back problems before she started the 13-week RunWalk program, Anna didn't think they would affect her efforts to complete the sessions. As it turns out, the then-35-year-old recreation therapist was painfully wrong. About six weeks in, one of her knees became unable to compensate for the alignment problems that started in her back. "I was totally devastated," she recalls. "I thought running just wasn't my sport."

She was going to quit the program altogether, but instead for a few weeks changed to the walking program (see SportMedBC's *Walking for Fitness: The Beginner's Guide*) and visited a physiotherapist, who got her swimming and cycling to strengthen the knee. "I went back to the RunWalk program in about three weeks. Although I was used to being at the front of the running pack when I first started, I had to get used to the idea of pulling up the rear, but I didn't mind at all. I found myself with all the people who joined the program for social reasons, thinking, hey if we finish it, great. They were really supportive."

Anna completed the running program with her original group and went on to complete a 10-k race in 1:20.

If you're lucky enough to live in a climate that's neither too hot nor too cold, you want to avoid overdressing. Your body will heat up when you run, and a jacket that's cozy when you start out will feel suffocating when you reach running temperature. When you overheat, you tend to lose a lot of body fluid through sweat, thereby dehydrating yourself. It's a good idea to layer clothes so that you can adjust the layers to suit weather conditions. You will quickly discover that a sweat-soaked cotton T-shirt plastered to your body feels as unpleasant as it looks.

In the last 10 years, there have been tremendous improvements in running and exercise clothing. Today, technical athletic clothing is primarily made of synthetic fibers, and you can find lightweight running shirts, sports bras, shorts and tights made from multiple layers of nylon- and polyester-based materials. According to LadySport's Phil Moore, "The weaves and textures of these fabrics are designed to wick moisture away from the skin, rather than absorbing it into the garment itself. Cotton, on the other hand, can absorb up to seven times its weight in water, resulting in clothing that is colder in winter, warmer in summer and very heavy when wet. Cotton also fades, stretches and shrinks." As well, says Moore, "The new materials use hydrophilic/hydrophobic layers, magnet technology, even silver or copper fibers to move moisture, manage temperature, increase breathability and reduce odor. Natural materials like merino wool are also great for wicking moisture and reducing unwanted odor! All of these improvements make running in any temperature and climate easier and more enjoyable."

Female runners will probably want to consider a sports bra, as physical activity causes the breasts to bounce. The breast is supported by a fragile structure of skin and ligaments that can be stretched by bouncing, leading to breast sag. Most everyday bras will not stop this bouncing. Enter the sports bra. Today's sports bras are well designed and

FACT

Cotton may be 100 percent natural, but it's not a fiber you want next to your body when you're sweating because it holds in moisture. Instead look for synthetic fabrics that wick moisture away from your body.

SUMMARY

> Start slowly. Follow the training schedule!

> Go at your own pace. Don't be pressured to run or walk faster than you are comfortable with.

> Think positively. Focus on what feels good, not on what hurts.

> Make time to work out. Set aside a specific time for your workouts and protect this time so that other commitments don't interfere with your training.

> Congratulate yourself. After a workout, stop and think about how good you feel. Remember this feeling the next time you're not too keen about heading out.

even serve as outerwear, making them a great option in hot weather. Look for a snug fit (to control motion) and a design that minimizes movement within the bra (to eliminate chafing). Large-breasted women should look for molded cups; smaller-breasted women can go with the compression-type bras that flatten the breasts. Avoid cups with seams that can irritate the nipple, and make sure any hardware is adequately cushioned. You'll want wide straps, because all that motion can make narrow straps slip off the shoulders. Many models now come with adjustable straps to help customize the fit. Finally, be sure your arms have enough room to move freely.

Again, be sure to wear some type of moisture-management material, regardless of the brand name; it's NO to cotton and YES to synthetics if the layer is right against your body!

Many people love running in the cold because it helps keep body temperature down, and some days it seems one could run forever. Still, you don't want to get too cold. Outerwear should be made of a breathable, waterproof fabric such as Gore-Tex (which is still the "gold standard" among fabrics on the market). Keep in mind that no matter how breathable the fabric, if you work up enough of a sweat you will overwhelm its ability to dissipate the moisture. A raised collar will help protect your neck, which can be especially sensitive in the cold; consider wearing a turtleneck. Layering is key! Keep a fitted moisture-management garment against your skin to avoid air pockets that can cool you down. Then, layer looser-fitting synthetics, lightweight fleece and rainproof clothing on top, depending on the temperature and rain conditions. And since as much as 70 percent of body heat is lost through your head, consider a hat, too. Gloves can keep your hands from feeling like they're freezing solid. If you wear socks (some runners don't), look for a fabric that will wick away moisture. Some runners avoid blistering by wearing two pairs of thin socks, or one pair of double-layer socks, that can rub against each other instead of against sensitive skin.

SETTING GOALS

People successful in any area of life, including sports and careers, share one common characteristic—they set realistic and meaningful goals for themselves. No one can safely compete in a 10-k event one week after they begin training.

Your mind, like your body, has to adjust to new levels of effort. If you set unrealistic goals for yourself and fail to achieve them, you will almost certainly become discouraged and perhaps quit. Why not set realistic goals to begin with and train your mind the same way you train your body? In the 13-week RunWalk program, the goals are set out for you, and the program is tried and true. Make a commitment to follow it, and you will likely succeed.

This doesn't mean you won't have lapses of confidence or motivation as you progress through the program. Becoming a runner takes the kind of effort against which most of our minds and bodies are inclined to rebel. But the 13-week program is designed to train your mind at the same time as it trains your body, so that you can face and move past the inevitable trials.

CHAPTER 2 SUMMARY

1. Remember the three basic rules of training: moderation, consistency and rest.
2. When choosing running shoes, visit a running store, have the staff assess your feet and help you choose a shoe that fits properly and suits your biomechanics.
3. Select a running jacket in cool weather and shirts, shorts and socks made from synthetic materials, which wick moisture and keep you dry.
4. For best success in your running program, start slowly, go at your own pace, think positively and congratulate yourself after each session.

PAR-Q & YOU

(A Questionnaire for People Aged 15 to 69)

Regular physical activity is fun and healthy, and increasingly more people are starting to become more active every day. Being more active is very safe for most people. However, some people should check with their doctor before they start becoming much more physically active.

If you are planning to become much more physically active than you are now, start by answering the seven questions in the box below. If you are between the ages of 15 and 69, the PAR-Q will tell you if you should check with your doctor before you start. If you are over 69 years of age, and you are not used to being very active, check with your doctor.

Common sense is your best guide when you answer these questions. Please read the questions carefully and answer each one honestly: check YES or NO.

YES	NO		
☐	☐	1.	**Has your doctor ever said that you have a heart condition <u>and</u> that you should only do physical activity recommended by a doctor?**
☐	☐	2.	**Do you feel pain in your chest when you do physical activity?**
☐	☐	3.	**In the past month, have you had chest pain when you were not doing physical activity?**
☐	☐	4.	**Do you lose your balance because of dizziness or do you ever lose consciousness?**
☐	☐	5.	**Do you have a bone or joint problem (for example, back, knee or hip) that could be made worse by a change in your physical activity?**
☐	☐	6.	**Is your doctor currently prescribing drugs (for example, water pills) for your blood pressure or heart condition?**
☐	☐	7.	**Do you know of <u>any other reason</u> why you should not do physical activity?**

If you answered

YES to one or more questions

Talk with your doctor by phone or in person BEFORE you start becoming much more physically active or BEFORE you have a fitness appraisal. Tell your doctor about the PAR-Q and which questions you answered YES.

- You may be able to do any activity you want — as long as you start slowly and build up gradually. Or, you may need to restrict your activities to those which are safe for you. Talk with your doctor about the kinds of activities you wish to participate in and follow his/her advice.
- Find out which community programs are safe and helpful for you.

NO to all questions

If you answered NO honestly to <u>all</u> PAR-Q questions, you can be reasonably sure that you can;
- start becoming much more physically active — begin slowly and build up gradually. This is the safest and easiest way to go.
- take part in a fitness appraisal — this is an excellent way to determine your basic fitness so that you can plan the best way for you to live actively. It is also highly recommended that you have your blood pressure evaluated. If your reading is over 144/94, talk with your doctor before you start becoming much more physically active.

DELAY BECOMING MUCH MORE ACTIVE:
- if you are not feeling well because of a temporary illness such as a cold or a fever — wait until you feel better; or
- if you are or may be pregnant — talk to your doctor before you start becoming more active.

PLEASE NOTE: If your health changes so that you then answer YES to any of the above questions, tell your fitness or health professional. Ask whether you should change your physical activity plan.

<u>Informed Use of the PAR-Q</u>: The Canadian Society for Exercise Physiology, Health Canada, and their agents assume no liability for persons who undertake physical activity, and if in doubt after completing this questionnaire, consult your doctor prior to physical activity.

No changes permitted. You are encouraged to photocopy the PAR-Q but only if you use the entire form.

NOTE: If the PAR-Q is being given to a person before he or she participates in a physical activity program or a fitness appraisal, this section may be used for legal or administrative purposes.

"I have read, understood and completed this questionnaire. Any questions I had were answered to my full satisfaction."

NAME _____

SIGNATURE _____ DATE_____

SIGNATURE OF PARENT _____ WITNESS _____
or GUARDIAN (for participants under the age of majority)

Note: This physical activity clearance is valid for a maximum of 12 months from the date it is completed and becomes invalid if your condition changes so that you would answer YES to any of the seven questions.

 CSEP | SCPE   © Canadian Society for Exercise Physiology www.csep.ca/forms

3

On the Road

....

THE 13-WEEK RUNWALK program is a template for fitness that has been used successfully by thousands of people to prepare for one of the largest running/walking events in North America, the *Vancouver Sun* Run™. The training schedule you will follow (page 44) starts off slowly to help you build strength, stamina and confidence. Your focus over the next 13 weeks will be to improve your overall health and fitness while remaining injury free. If possible, find a friend or a group of friends to train with you. It's not only more fun with friends, it's also more motivating.

Each training session is broken down into short RunWalk blocks. These blocks are long enough to lead to improvement but not so onerous that you will feel exhausted or sore. There's a psychological benefit as well: the tasks in each block are relatively easy to complete, which will give you the confidence to go on.

Study the program carefully to see where you will be going and how long it will take you to get there. It's important to remember that the times noted for the training sessions also include the time you will have to spend warming up and cooling down, five minutes at either end of the training session. As the weeks pass, the ratio of running to walking increases, until by the last week you are just running.

However, you will notice a new RunWalk option provided after Week 6. At that point you will be encouraged to reflect on how your body is adapting to the training and, if you are struggling, you will have the option of continuing to RunWalk for the remaining weeks. You will still be prepared to cover the 10-k distance, but you will RunWalk it as opposed to running only. As early as the second or third week, you may start to feel quite comfortable with the workouts and may feel ready to jump ahead. But your bones, ligaments, tendons and muscles adapt to training much less quickly than your cardio-vascular system; to stay injury free, you must give them time to catch up. Getting injured halfway through the program would be far more discouraging than taking the prescribed time to get to the continuous running stage.

Schedule enough time each week to complete the three training sessions with rest days in between, rather than trying to squeeze your training sessions into consecutive days. Many people find it helps to start on a weekend. It also helps to pick a running route that's enticing, and as free of obstacles—pedestrians and cars—as possible. Think of running an "out-and-back route," and at the halfway point, head back home.

One piece of equipment you will definitely need is a sport watch with a stopwatch feature. Digital is best; sweep second-hand readings tend to get approximated when you're bouncing along.

KEEPING A TRAINING LOG

Many fitness enthusiasts keep training logs, and athletes often have daily training records going back 10 years or more. These records allow them to see the big picture, the patterns that emerge only over time. If you decide to keep a training log, you may find it a hassle at first, but if you keep detailed notes on such things as diet and sleep patterns, how much time you spent warming up and stretching, and when, where and how far you ran, it will allow you to see a new, healthier pattern starting to form in your life.

You may find you even start recording your thoughts, a practice that can really pay dividends. Many runners say their moments of greatest clarity come when they are running, and you may find your insights worth recalling at a later date. At the very least, a year or two down the road you can look back at your old training logs and laugh when you see an entry describing how you maxed out at 545 yards (500 meters) of running—when today you can knock off 5 k without breaking a sweat. (Refer to Resources and References—page 207—for training log suggestions.)

Many people find that keeping a journal is motivating. If you're having a tough time getting up off the couch, try picking up your training log and flipping through the pages summarizing all your hard work. Then look at the next, blank page—the one that can't be filled in until after that day's training session. Most of the time this will be enough to get you lacing up your shoes.

Keeping a training log in which you record aches and pains can also help you to prevent injuries, or at least to better recover from them. Noting your aches and pains may motivate you to deal with their causes before they lead to actual injuries. And if you *do* become injured, the log will allow you to work more closely with your doctor or physiotherapist, detailing the kinds of problems you've been having and how they originally manifested.

In a nutshell, keeping a training log will enable you to
> analyze the effects of your training
> monitor your progress
> develop a systematic plan for improvement
> avoid overtraining and injury
> stay motivated
> look back in wonder, amusement or perhaps even amazement

FACT

Consider jotting down notes about your diet in your training log. Having a record of food intake can help you identify problem times, moods or stresses that affect your eating. And you'll be able to see how all these things affect your training.

WARMING UP

No matter how motivated you are, if running or brisk walking has not been part of your daily life, your body will find exercise something of a shock. The 13-week RunWalk program is designed to minimize the shock, but the need for warm-up exercises before every training session cannot be overemphasized. Warming up is not just for beginners—even world-class athletes need to warm up before every workout.

The purpose of a warm-up routine is to prepare your body for exercise. (Warming up itself should not be thought of as exercise, even if the routines are called warm-up "exercises.") Cold muscles work less efficiently and are more easily injured. They lack the flow of blood necessary to do the work called for by exercise.

Your warm-up should include some kind of general body movement designed to get the blood flowing. After about 10 minutes of moving your arms, legs and trunk continuously, you can proceed to some gentle stretching, and the accent here is on gentle. Wendy Epp, a sport physiotherapist and competitive runner and triathlete, points out that research shows you're more likely to pull a cold muscle by stretching too vigorously than by actually starting right into jogging. "It's important to warm up progressively. A low-intensity, rhythmic activity like gentle jogging, which takes your muscles through a limited range of motion, will increase muscle and body temperature gradually and thus minimize the risk of injury."

Epp offers a simple analogy. She compares muscles to plasticine, the children's toy you can mold into different shapes. When it's cold, plasticine is hard and brittle, so if you attack it with any degree of force, it tends to break rather than bend. Only after it has been gently kneaded and manipulated does it assume its malleable character. Your muscles respond in much the same way.

The rule with stretching, before, during and after exercise, is to listen to your body: if it hurts, you've gone too far. This is true no matter how fit you are or how fast you run. You might find it annoying to get a running injury, but just imagine how frustrated you'd feel if the injury resulted from something you thought you were doing to avoid being injured!

An array of running-specific stretches is provided on pages 182–91. Make these stretches part of every training session. In general, runners and walkers should focus on their calf, hamstring, gluteal, hip flexor and lower back muscles. Hold each stretch for about 10 seconds and repeat two to three times per muscle group.

A good warm-up routine

> Walk or jog slowly for five to 10 minutes.
> Stretch lightly for three to five minutes, concentrating on your calves, hamstrings, quadriceps, gluteals, hip flexors, lower back muscles and shoulders. (See exercises on pages 182–86.)

COOLING DOWN

Just as a warm-up is the best way to prepare your body for increased levels of activity, a cooling-down procedure is the best way to ease it back down to idle speed. It's a good idea to keep your muscles active for 10 to 15 minutes after exercising using a similar but less intense version of what you did during your warm-up. Light stretching is sufficient for your cool-down; hold each stretch for 15 to 30 seconds and repeat two to three times.

In time you'll find that the nice warm muscles you developed during your training session are more pliable, and that makes your post-exercise period a perfect time to work on your flexibility. After your training session has your muscles thoroughly warmed up, you can safely hold each stretch for anywhere from 30 seconds to three minutes.

Post-activity stretching serves two purposes. The most important reason you want to stretch after your training session is that muscles tighten during exercise, and unless you stretch them out again, they tend to stay tight.

The other benefit to cool-down stretching is that it can help you increase the range of motion in your joints. Keep in mind that your ability to increase your range of motion is influenced by a number of things, including age, pre-existing conditions (such as old injuries) and joint structure. Try not to think of stretching as a competitive sport. Every body stretches differently, and the fact that your running partner seems able to stretch farther doesn't mean there's something wrong with you. Be satisfied with incremental gains and look for benefits over the long haul.

Some athletes argue that post-exercise stretching is the key to avoiding muscle soreness, but the case has been overstated. A certain amount of muscle soreness is natural after exercise. If you don't find yourself back to normal in about

MICHAEL, 51, always found his running partner's insistence on warming up and cooling down an aggravation. Once his running shoes were laced up, the last thing he wanted to do was stand around stretching. "Once it's time to go, I just want to go. I hate waiting."

One night he awoke with his hamstrings locked up. "I couldn't believe the pain. I reached down and felt the muscle and it was like steel. I wanted to stretch out my leg but I couldn't. My wife woke up almost certain I was having a heart attack; I think I was screaming."

Luckily his wife had been a swimmer and knew all about cramps. She rolled him onto his back and used her entire body weight to push down on his knee while at the same time using both hands to pull his ankle. Eventually the muscle started to give, and the more it stretched out the more pliable it became, until Michael's leg was lying flat on the bed.

When I told my running partner about it, he just shook his head and told me to start thinking about post-run stretching. "Now I do it religiously. I still hate it but I only have to recall that night to get on with it."

48 hours, however, you may have injured yourself. If you think this may be the case, see a qualified sport medicine practitioner.

To sum up, begin your cool-down by walking or slowly jogging for five to 10 minutes. Then repeat your warm-up stretching routine, again paying special attention to stretches working your calves, hamstrings, gluteals, hip flexors and lower back muscles. For cool-down only, hold each stretch about 15 to 30 seconds, repeating two to three times per muscle group. If you are working on your flexibility, hold each stretch position for anywhere from 30 seconds to three minutes and repeat two to three times per muscle group.

A good cool-down routine

> Walk or jog slowly for five to 10 minutes, keeping your arms moving forward and back in circles.
> Stretch your hamstring and calf muscles for flexibility now that they are warm. (See exercises on page 183.)
> Stretch deeply only after you are completely warmed up—after your workout—to increase or maintain your level of flexibility.

RUNNING TECHNIQUES

When you first start running, technique will likely not be something you need worry about. Most bodies automatically adopt the technique best suited to them. (At least, they do so in the best of all possible worlds. The wrench in the works can be old injuries or hereditary misalignments. See Chapter 9, Common Injuries and Recovery.)

The amount of energy lost because of poor running technique becomes more of an issue when and if you start running longer distances. Running coach Roy Benson describes the ideal biomechanics of an elite runner as follows: "The key seems to be in watching the upper body and making sure the shoulders aren't overrotating, twisting from side to side. The arm swing should be just as comfortable as if you were walking, swinging a little bit away from you on the backside to just in front of your thigh in the front."

If you find this difficult to envisage, don't worry about your form—being relaxed is even more important. Although most people get tense when they're physically stressed, runners should avoid tension for at least two reasons. First, tight muscles may be more susceptible to injury. Second, it takes a lot of energy to stay tense; relaxing helps channel that energy into running. While you're following the 13-week program, just try to think about relaxing, assuming good posture (open up your chest cavity by not hunching forward) and putting one foot in front of the other. If you have problems you think might be caused by poor technique, see Chapter 7, Becoming a Better Runner, where running technique is examined in more detail.

SAFETY FIRST

Running alone can make you vulnerable, especially if you are a woman. With the view that forewarned is forearmed, here are a few safety tips to make your training sessions more enjoyable—by making them safer.

> Always carry identification or write your name, phone number and blood type on a piece of paper. Put it in a running shoe key holder and attach it to the top of one of your shoes.
> Carry appropriate coins in case you need to use the phone. Keep a whistle or noisemaker in your pocket or hanging around your neck.
> Don't wear jewelry—it can attract attention you really don't want.
> Write down your running route and leave it with a friend or somewhere it can easily be found. Discuss running routes with your running friends and family.
> Run in familiar areas. Know the location of telephones and businesses or stores that are sure to be open when you run. Don't be too predictable—consider altering your route every

now and again, especially if the same person frequently shows up on your route.

> Depending on where you live, <u>avoid running in unpopulated</u> areas, and on deserted streets and overgrown trails. Avoid <u>unlit</u> areas at night. Stay clear of parked cars and bushes.

> Run against traffic so you can observe approaching vehicles. Remember, your seeing the cars does not guarantee that their drivers see you. If they're coming up behind you, you're vulnerable.

> Respect the flow of traffic. Stay out of bicycle and vehicle lanes. Move out of the way when you are being passed by cyclists or in-line skaters on shared pathways. If you are running or walking in a group, go in single file, leave room for

---

CLARE never thought much about running technique. The 37-year-old never had any aches and pains from the sport and she never ran for more than 30 minutes at a time. However, she seemed to tire faster than her running partners.

Although she tended to slouch, Clare never thought her posture might be affecting her running. One day her training partner was massaging her neck after a training session and commented on its tightness. Her partner suggested that the tension and fatigue might stem from some kind of problem with her running technique, so Clare asked an instructor at her gym to watch her run. He told her that she <u>hunched over</u> and was <u>tensing up</u>, which might be contributing to the tight muscles. And because slouching can constrict the chest cavity and reduce lung capacity, it might be contributing to her fatigue. He told her to "<u>run tall</u>," to pull back her shoulders and lift her chin.

"It's not like a miracle cure or anything," Clare says, "but once I started to think about my posture and my running technique, I started to think about it all the time. Now I really do think my posture and breathing are better."

Clare

others to get by and keep an eye open for pedestrians and small children.

> If you're running in low light or after dark, wear clothing with reflective strips. If you don't like any of the gear that comes with such strips, buy some reflective tape and put it on the clothing you do like to wear. Consider a reflective vest. Ankle reflectors designed for cyclists work just as well for runners.

> Stay alert. The more aware you are of your surroundings, the less vulnerable you are and the greater the likelihood that you will be prepared to act in an emergency. For this reason, don't wear headphones when you train. Your ears are a survival tool, a kind of 360-degree aural radar. Don't defeat their purpose.

> Ignore verbal harassment. Use discretion in acknowledging strangers. Look directly at people and be observant, but keep your distance and keep moving.

> Trust your intuition. Avoid any person or area that "feels" unsafe.

> Call the police immediately if something happens to you or someone else, or if you are being followed or harassed.

ADAPTING TO THE WEATHER

You can run any time of the year: all you need is the proper gear, the right preparation and a positive attitude. In the summer, the biggest challenge to runners is the heat. In the winter, cold temperatures, wet snow and slippery conditions can all be deterrents to lacing up your runners and hitting the pavement. But no matter the climate, you can still run. In fact, one of the great pleasures of running can be observing the changes in your favorite running route at different times of day, over the seasons and in variable weather conditions.

Hot-weather running

The best way to acclimate to hot-weather running is to do it gradually, wearing the proper clothing and staying hydrated.

Keep in mind that your body needs to work harder to cool you down by producing sweat. Listen to your body and remember the following tips:

> Slow down and/or shorten your run.
> Protect yourself from the sun by wearing a mesh hat and applying sunblock.
> Wear a light-colored or white shirt made of synthetic material; it will keep you cool by moving sweat away from your body.
> Drink more water than usual before, during and after a run.
> Run at cooler times of the day, such as in the early morning or in the evening.
> Plan a route that takes you through a kids' water park or along shady forest trails.

Cold-weather running

Some people love to run in the cold because it gives them more energy. Be especially vigilant if conditions are icy or wet, and remember that snowy surfaces provide better traction than icy roads. Hypothermia and frostbite are two dangers you may face when running in the cold, so it's especially important to dress in layers and protect your head, face and fingers. Here are some tips for cold-weather running:

> If there is ice on the road, slow down your run so you don't get injured.
> Keep warm by including a hat, gloves and a windbreaker as part of your gear.
> Layer your clothes so you can better regulate your body temperature.
> Keep moving; standing still will cause you to cool down quickly.
> Run on forest trails, which can protect you from the wind and rain.

CHAPTER 3 SUMMARY

1. Keep a training log to monitor your progress, keep you motivated and help prevent injuries.
2. Before your run, spend five minutes warming up so you don't strain your muscles when you begin your workout.
3. After your run, spend five minutes gently stretching to loosen up your muscles and improve your flexibility.
4. Stay relaxed: concentrate on standing tall and swinging your arms naturally as you run.
5. Stay alert and keep safety in mind whenever and wherever you run.

4

Let's Get Started
The 13-Week RunWalk
Program

....

The Beginning Runner's Handbook includes everything you need to be successful at learning to run a 10 k. Previous chapters have armed you with some basic principles that lay the foundation for your training, and later chapters provide important information and direction on stretching exercises for warm-ups and cool-downs and strength-training exercises to complement your running program. This chapter provides detailed weekly training plans along with coaching advice and useful tips. Using all of these elements together, you are just weeks away from achieving a new level of fitness.

Proper warm-up, cool-down and stretching exercises are essential if you want to avoid injury. The recommended stretches outlined in Appendix A are a key part of your training program, and Chapter 3 provided some details on how, when and how much you should be stretching before and after your training sessions. Don't try to save time by eliminating these important components of your training sessions.

Most successful athletes keep a training log. There are a variety of running logbooks or journals to choose from (see Resources and References, pages 208 and 209), and over time you will develop your own style of record keeping. Setting realistic and meaningful goals will help you progress through each week of training.

THE 13-WEEK PROGRAM

The SportMed RunWalk program is a carefully tested exercise plan that involves three training sessions each week, ranging in length from 28 to 76 minutes. It is important that you spread out these training sessions evenly throughout the week and try to develop a fixed schedule.

You'll notice that the program starts gradually, with lots of walking. A sport watch can help you time the RunWalk segments of your sessions. If you find the progressions too slow, bear with the program and don't be tempted to skip ahead. You won't increase your fitness—just your risk of injury. One of the most significant updates to the training program is the RunWalk option, which allows those who have been struggling through the first six weeks to take a more gradual approach to the end of the program. You will still be preparing to cover the 10-k distance but with RunWalk intervals rather than running the entire way.

The "run" portion of your training should be a very slow jog, always at a comfortable talking pace. You should feel as though you could walk briskly as fast as you are running and you should be able to carry on a conversation, two or three sentences at a time, without losing your breath. In the beginning, excitement and anxiety about your workouts can cause you to run at a quicker pace than you can handle. Pay attention to your speed: as the pace increases so does the impact and the likelihood of incurring an injury.

Remember, running is not easy. It takes time for muscles, tendons, bones and ligaments to adapt to the impact. If you stick to the program, doing no more and no less, you'll be surprised how easy it will be. Finally, note that the workout times include your five-minute warm-up and five-minute cool-down in each training session. Be sure to incorporate these essential components into your schedule.

WEEK 1: It's All about Pace

☐ **Session 1** (34 minutes)
Run one minute. Walk two minutes.
Do this eight times.

☐ **Session 2** (28 minutes)
Run one minute. Walk two minutes.
Do this six times.

☐ **Session 3** (31 minutes)
Run one minute. Walk two minutes.
Do this seven times.

TIP

For runners, the most important piece of equipment is a good pair of supportive running shoes. You will also want to have clothing, especially the layers next to the skin, made of synthetic fabrics that wick moisture away from your body.

COACHING ADVICE

In order to ease your way into running, use the "shuffle-jog" technique—stand tall, use a short arm swing and take little steps without lifting your knees. Try not to bounce; this is intended to be a shuffle. (Picture a boxer training with short punchy arms and quick-action shuffle steps, or even a dancer doing the cha-cha.) Distribute your weight over the middle to front of your foot, unlike walking, which is clearly a heel-toe action. Your transition from walking to running and vice versa should be so smooth that your body and mind hardly know the difference.

It is important to find
the time to include all
three training sessions
each week. The program
progresses as the weeks
go by and, in order to be
successful, you need to
"do your homework." If
you are unable to com-
plete the week for any
reason, consider repeat-
ing it and then carrying
on from there.

WEEK 2: Building the Foundation

☐ **Session 1** (38 minutes)
Run two minutes. Walk two minutes.
Do this seven times.

☐ **Session 2** (31 minutes)
Run one minute. Walk two minutes.
Do this seven times.

☐ **Session 3** (34 minutes)
Run two minutes. Walk two minutes.
Do this six times.

COACHING ADVICE

You likely found last week's one-minute shuffle-jogs fairly easy. If you kept the pace slow and easy, you may even have felt frustrated by the minimal effort. This week, try completing a couple of the two-minute repeats of running on the spot, to remind yourself of how it feels to maintain an easy and relaxed pace. Remember the shuffle-jog technique we introduced last week.

WEEK 3: Increasing Your Time Running

☐ **Session 1** (45 minutes)
Run three minutes. Walk two minutes.
Do this seven times.

☐ **Session 2** (34 minutes)
Run two minutes. Walk two minutes.
Do this six times.

☐ **Session 3** (40 minutes)
Run three minutes. Walk two minutes.
Do this six times.

COACHING ADVICE

As the running portion of the session gets longer, remember it's the arm swing that regulates your rhythm and pace. Try to keep your shoulders square and relaxed. Drive your arms comfortably backward and allow them to swing forward freely, keeping your elbows tucked into your sides. This will help you maintain a comfortable rhythm. Your legs will adjust accordingly. As your body adapts and your fitness improves, longer strides and a faster pace will come naturally, but for now, it's all about your personal rhythm and pace.

TIP

Keep a record of your progress in a training journal. Maintaining a logbook will help you track the origin of any injuries. Note how you feel each session, when and where you train, what is going on in your life (were you up all night before your run with sick kids, for example) and anything else that you feel like jotting down. This is the best way to set your goals and monitor your progress. Remember to keep it simple and be honest!

Always try to think posi-
tively. Focus on what
feels good, not on what
hurts. At the beginning
of the program, vari-
ous aches and pains will
develop as your body
begins to adapt to the
new stress levels. Be
patient; this is all part of
the process.

WEEK 4: Easy Recovery Week

☐ **Session 1** (40 minutes)
Run three minutes. Walk two minutes.
Do this six times.

☐ **Session 2** (30 minutes)
Run two minutes. Walk two minutes.
Do this five times.

☐ **Session 3** (40 minutes)
Run two minutes. Walk three minutes.
Do this six times.

COACHING ADVICE

You've already come a long way since Week 1, and your body needs a bit of
a rest as you slowly build your fitness. Remember how unsure of yourself
you were when you first tackled these running intervals? You should now
be familiar with your own comfort zone and have more confidence with
your rhythm and pace. Enjoy this "easy" week, and keep your pace relaxed
and comfortable.

WEEK 5: Focusing on Your "Shuffle"

☐ **Session 1** (46 minutes)
Run three minutes. Walk one minute.
Do this nine times.

☐ **Session 2** (34 minutes)
Run two minutes. Walk one minute.
Do this eight times.

☐ **Session 3** (42 minutes)
Run three minutes. Walk one minute.
Do this eight times.

TIP

Search out an exercise partner who will make the 13-week training commitment with you. It sure helps to know that someone is on the corner waiting for you—and it's incredible how you can push and pull each other through a training session.

COACHING ADVICE

After last week's "recovery," you shouldn't have any problem with the three-minute shuffle-jogging intervals this week. The big difference now is that your walk (recovery) time is reduced to a minute, which will go by quickly, so it's more important than ever to run at a shuffle pace. If you feel like you are huffin' and puffin' and clearly not running at talking pace, you must slow down.

TIP

......
TIP
......

If you are experiencing a few aches and pains, "ice them." Fill Styrofoam cups with water and freeze them. When you want to ice an aching body part before and/or after your workout, simply peel back the Styrofoam and apply.

WEEK 6: Increasing Your Workload

☐ **Session 1** (52 minutes)
Run five minutes. Walk one minute. Do this seven times.

☐ **Session 2** (38 minutes)
Run three minutes. Walk one minute. Do this seven times.

☐ **Session 3** (50 minutes)
Run three minutes. Walk one minute. Do this 10 times.

COACHING ADVICE

At this stage, you may be starting to feel tired. Although it's tempting to take a break, persevere and you should start to feel better soon. This is a good time to take a break from the roads and search out a softer surface, grass or trail. The new terrain will provide your legs with a much-needed reprieve from the pavement and a change of scenery. Hang in there; the tiredness will subside. Remember to monitor your pace and slow down if necessary to avoid injury.

MIDWAY CHECK-IN!

The end goal of the 13-week program is for you to safely and comfortably complete a 10-k distance. Now that you are half-way through the program, this is a good time to assess how you are feeling. Be honest with yourself and understand that everyone responds to training differently. If the running segments have been comfortable, then continue on with the program progressions. Your running time will continue to increase with significantly less walking time in between. By the end of the 13 weeks, you will be prepared to run the entire 10-k distance with very little, if any, walking.

If you have been struggling to complete the running segments or simply like the idea of staying with a combination of running and walking, choose the RunWalk option that we have included from this point on. You will still be prepared at the end of the 13 weeks to complete the 10-k distance; however, you will be running and walking as opposed to running only. In fact, your run segments will never exceed 10 minutes and are always followed by a short walking segment.

The key is to feel comfortable throughout the program: know that you can always choose the RunWalk option presented each week, depending on how you are feeling.

Pace your training ses-
sion on windy days by
running *into* the wind
when you start and
still have lots of energy.
Come home with the
wind at your back.

WEEK 7: Over Halfway There

☐ **Session 1** (54 minutes or 5-k distance)
Run 10 minutes. Walk one minute.
Do this four times or repeat pattern over the 5-k distance.

☐ **Session 2** (40 minutes)
Run four minutes. Walk one minute. Do this six times.

☐ **Session 3** (52 minutes)
Run five minutes. Walk one minute. Do this seven times.

RunWalk Option

☐ **Session 1** (52 minutes or 5-k distance)
Run six minutes. Walk one minute.
Do this six times or repeat pattern over the 5-k distance.

☐ **Session 2** (40 minutes)
Run four minutes. Walk one minute. Do this six times.

☐ **Session 3** (50 minutes)
Run four minutes. Walk one minute. Do this eight times.

COACHING ADVICE

Congratulations! You are over halfway through the program, and you have
learned so much about what your body can handle. In the remaining weeks,
you will have the RunWalk option available to you, and you can choose it
at any time. This week, boost your confidence and test yourself over a 5-k
distance. Find an appropriate place to mark out a reasonably accurate 5-k
course and perform your prescribed workout over that route. Remember
to stay relaxed and keep the pace consistent as always. Focus on your arm
action, and the legs will follow.

WEEK 8: Easy Recovery Week

☐ **Session 1** (54 minutes)
Run 10 minutes. Walk one minute. Do this four times.

☐ **Session 2** (38 minutes)
Run three minutes. Walk one minute. Do this seven times.

☐ **Session 3** (46 minutes)
Run five minutes. Walk one minute. Do this six times.

RunWalk Option

☐ **Session 1** (52 minutes)
Run five minutes. Walk one minute. Do this seven times.

☐ **Session 2** (38 minutes)
Run three minutes. Walk one minute. Do this seven times.

☐ **Session 3** (46 minutes)
Run two minutes. Walk one minute. Do this 12 times.

You've reached another important milestone in your 13-week program: every fourth week in the program is a well-earned recovery week, and this week's plateau is a good week to take a break, especially if you have any unusual aches or pains. Try replacing one session with some low-impact cross training, such as "running" your intervals in the deep end of a pool to give your legs a rest but still keep some cardio training.

TIP

Pool running can be far less tedious than swimming laps. Do it with a friend—you can talk like you're on a jog. To pass the time, alternate slow and fast efforts. Pick a pool that plays good tunes and run to the music!

COACHING ADVICE

WEEK 9: Back to Work

☐ **Session 1** (68 minutes)
Run 10 minutes. Walk one minute.
Run 15 minutes. Walk one minute.
Run 20 minutes. Walk one minute.
Run 10 minutes.

☐ **Session 2** (46 minutes)
Run five minutes. Walk one minute. Do this six times.

☐ **Session 3** (54 minutes)
Run 10 minutes. Walk one minute. Do this four times.

RunWalk Option

☐ **Session 1** (66 minutes)
Run six minutes. Walk one minute. Do this eight times.

☐ **Session 2** (45 minutes)
Run four minutes. Walk one minute. Do this seven times.

☐ **Session 3** (55 minutes)
Run four minutes. Walk one minute. Do this nine times.

COACHING ADVICE

It's time to get back to business. After an easy recovery week, you're ready to increase your workload again. This week, you'll face steady increases in running time and total workout time, but you are ready for it. Stay confident, strong and relaxed. Let your arms control your rhythm and, above all, keep the pace slow and at a talking pace. The walk portions are now simply a mental break for you.

WEEK 10: A Big Week

☐ **Session 1** (72 minutes)
Run 10 minutes. Walk one minute.
Run 20 minutes. Walk one minute.
Run 30 minutes.

☐ **Session 2** (54 minutes)
Run 10 minutes. Walk one minute. Do this four times.

☐ **Session 3** (57 minutes)
Run 20 minutes. Walk one minute.
Run 15 minutes. Walk one minute.
Run 10 minutes.

RunWalk Option

☐ **Session 1** (73 minutes)
Run eight minutes. Walk one minute. Do this seven times.

☐ **Session 2** (55 minutes)
Run four minutes. Walk one minute. Do this nine times.

☐ **Session 3** (58 minutes)
Run five minutes. Walk one minute. Do this eight times.

Listen to your body. Pay attention to what it's telling you. If you are sick with a cold or flu, take a day or two off from training. Give yourself a chance to recover before resuming your workouts.

COACHING ADVICE

This is a big week as you spend more time running, though with the usual minute of walking between intervals. You are ready for it: focus on a relaxed, comfortable arm action to maintain your rhythm. Remember, although you might like to go faster, "speed" is truly irrelevant right now. This part of the program is all about getting used to impact and distance, and it's usually the toughest for most people. Stay motivated and fight through the fatigue by smiling. It's contagious, and you'll feel great when someone smiles back!

Work at staying healthy
and injury free. Take care
of your health by getting
enough sleep, eating
balanced meals and
staying hydrated. Keep a
water bottle with you at
all times and sip from it
throughout the day.

WEEK 11: Building Confidence

☐ **Session 1** (71 minutes)
Run 40 minutes. Walk one minute.
Run 20 minutes.

☐ **Session 2** (54 minutes)
Run 10 minutes. Walk one minute. Do this four times.

☐ **Session 3** (57 minutes)
Run 20 minutes. Walk one minute.
Run 15 minutes. Walk one minute.
Run 10 minutes.

RunWalk Option

☐ **Session 1** (76 minutes)
Run 10 minutes. Walk one minute. Do this six times.

☐ **Session 2** (55 minutes)
Run 4 minutes. Walk one minute. Do this nine times.

☐ **Session 3** (58 minutes)
Run five minutes. Walk one minute. Do this eight times.

COACHING ADVICE

You will need your enthusiasm more than ever now as you reach your maximums in both volume and total running time this week. Providing you stay within your own personal talking pace, you are now able to run as long as you need to complete the 10 k! If you are doing the RunWalk option, you're running for 10 minutes at a time and have reached a milestone 76 minutes in workout time. Whichever option you've chosen, you are now running much longer than you're walking.

WEEK 12: Easy Volume Week

☐ **Session 1** (60 minutes)
Run 50 minutes.

☐ **Session 2** (43 minutes)
Run 10 minutes. Walk one minute. Do this three times.

☐ **Session 3** (52 minutes)
Run 15 minutes. Walk one minute.
Run 15 minutes. Walk one minute.
Run 10 minutes.

RunWalk Option

☐ **Session 1** (64 minutes)
Run eight minutes. Walk one minute. Do this six times.

☐ **Session 2** (40 minutes)
Run four minutes. Walk one minute. Do this six times.

☐ **Session 3** (52 minutes)
Run five minutes. Walk one minute. Do this seven times.

COACHING ADVICE

You're almost there! This is a very important recovery week. Mentally, imagine yourself completing the 10 k or, for those of you entering a 10-k event, crossing the finish line. You *can* do it. At this stage, resist the temptation to "test yourself" over the race course you will be running. Have confidence in your preparation and save your best for event day. If you really must assess whether or not you can go the distance, do only 8 k and leave yourself feeling great and wanting to do more.

WEEK 13: Congratulations!

☐ **Session 1** (50 minutes)
Run 40 minutes.

☐ **Session 2** (43 minutes)
Run 10 minutes. Walk one minute. Do this three times.

☐ **Session 3**
10 k: Run as you feel, have fun and take care not to start out too quickly.

RunWalk Option

☐ **Session 1** (54 minutes)
Run 10 minutes. Walk one minute. Do this four times.

☐ **Session 2** (40 minutes)
Run four minutes. Walk one minute. Do this six times.

☐ **Session 3**
10 k: RunWalk as you feel, have fun and take care not to start out too quickly.

COACHING ADVICE

You are ready to safely and comfortably complete your 10-k distance, either running or RunWalking. Have great confidence in your preparation: the hard work is done, and it's time for the grand finale. This is a nice easy week to allow your muscles and mind a full recovery so that you feel rested and ready. You did it!

Technique

> Walking and jogging are the most natural things we do, but our individual technique is unique.
> Your own personal running technique will evolve as you get stronger and, possibly, if you incorporate a few running exercises into the program to develop strength.
> Remember, use your arms when walking or jogging; your arms dictate your pace.
> If you consciously think about your arm action, your leg action will follow.

Avoiding side "stitches" (cramps) and tension

> Alter your breathing pattern by exhaling forcefully (grunt on exhalation).
> Belly breathe (breathe mainly with your diaphragm).
> Increase your core (abdominal) strength through exercises.
> Pinch together your thumb and middle finger to relax your shoulders and take the stress out of your upper body by concentrating on this small pressure point.

To complement the 13-week RunWalk program,

> continue to run or RunWalk three times a week
> join a running or walking club
> sign up for running or walking events—check your local running shoe store or community center
> keep an exercise/activity log to record your workouts
> try other activities—cycling, swimming and hiking are just a few of the numerous, excellent alternatives to running
> check out Chapter 11 for more great ideas

5

The Psychology
of Running

....

RUNNERS COME to appreciate early in their running careers that a
fit body won't travel very far if there isn't a fit mind traveling along
with it. Sometime during your training—probably on a cold, rainy,
windswept day—you may find yourself staring out the window and
discover that you have a remarkable capacity for making excuses.
You'll be able to come up with all sorts of reasons to avoid heading
out into what has suddenly become a world hostile to running. Or
perhaps it's not that hostile, but you're just not in the mood. In this
mind game, the solitary player is both winner and loser. You win by
avoiding what you don't want to do; you lose by avoiding what you
know needs to be done.

Staying on track is sometimes more difficult than initially getting to it. The 13-week RunWalk program is designed to help you
become a runner while exposing you to the least amount of risk,
both physical and mental. However, running is work. Getting
your heart rate up and covering increasing distances will make
you sweat and tire you out. Your body and mind will benefit, but
the action itself will be laborious. For that reason, as you progress

through the program, and even later on when you've trained yourself to be a runner, there may be days when you just don't feel like running. This chapter offers suggestions for dealing with those days.

LISTEN TO YOUR BODY

Sometimes you should listen to your body and not run. If you're sick, subjecting your body to additional stress might lead to injury or more serious illness. Your body needs its strength to recover; give it a chance. This includes times when you made yourself sick in the first place, by staying out too late, eating too much or drinking too much alcohol. (A lot of people think the best cure for a hangover is strenuous physical exercise, but this probably has more to do with a desire for self-punishment than the benefits of exercise. Avoid the problem in the first place by not overindulging.)

The same goes for running when you have a minor injury, or one that could become serious if not attended to. Some athletes are constantly nursing chronic aches and pains; yet many other athletes almost never seem to suffer from long-term disabilities. If you ask both how they deal with injuries, you will almost invariably learn that the chronically injured ones think it's nobler to run through pain than to take a break or deal with the problem. "Ignore it long enough and it will go away," they'll often tell you.

They're nearly always wrong.

TRAIN YOUR MIND

Motivation is a funny thing. You've probably found that you have more of it when you're not actually confronting whatever task you have assigned yourself. Napoleon understood this when he spoke of "the courage of the early morning." Soldiers would boast around the campfires at night, when they had some wine in their bellies, but were often less brave when the sun appeared on the horizon and the time came to march into battle. The truly brave, said Napoleon, were those whose courage did not abandon them when they strapped on their cuirasses and mounted their steeds.

The same is true for athletes. It's easy to conquer mountains or run marathons when the lights are out and you're peacefully dozing under the blankets; it's quite another when you're awake. To go from being a dreamer to being a doer, you have to train your mind the same way you train your body.

Nobody says, "I'm going to be a runner," and a month or two later jogs across the finish line at the New York Marathon. To become a runner, you train your body slowly, over an extended period. If you stick with the program in this book, you will develop a more robust cardiovascular system and a toughened musculoskeletal system, and you will be able to

RUNNER PROFILE

Chris

AFTER 40 years of inertia, Chris found himself wondering about the state of his health as he struggled through his middle years. The 64-year-old operator of a chain of retail gift stores decided to join a running clinic. "It was a little intimidating at first; there were hardly any other guys as old as I was. But when the program started out so slowly, I found I was okay.

His heightened level of fitness had a positive effect on his marriage, he adds. While his wife hasn't taken up running, she started in-line skating and now skates beside him as he pants his way through local parks.

Motivation is a problem for him now and then, but he's already figured out that if the spirit is unwilling, the best thing to do is call up a friend and rely on the buddy system. "Some of the rainy nights can be tough, but I find the best thing is to go with other people and not to try to do it by yourself. That's the whole secret for me; I always maintain that if you try to do it all yourself, you'll never make it."

run for some distance without gasping for air or pulling an Achilles tendon.

Your mind, too, needs training. You don't go from thinking on Tuesday that runners are lunatics to motivating yourself to run 30 minutes on Wednesday. Train your mind the same way you train your body: moderately, consistently and with the reward of rest for its efforts. If you do these things, your mind will serve your goals instead of sabotaging them.

Think of yourself as an athlete

Your first and most important goal for the mind is to think of yourself as an athlete. No matter how far you can run, you are an athlete. No matter what your reason for taking up running—whether it's weight control, overall fitness, social contacts or something else—you are an athlete. You subject yourself to regular training sessions and stress both your mind and body in pursuit of your goals, so you are, by definition, an athlete. It may seem like an exaggeration, but once you lace on a good pair of running shoes, you are—if you'll pardon the pun—on an equal footing with the world's best runners. "Oh sure," you say, "like I could run with the world's best!" In fact, you can. If you were to line up at the London Marathon, for example, you'd be toe to toe with the world's premier runners, on the same surface, using the same equipment. You might lose sight of them pretty quickly and not see them again for several hours, but unlike just about any other sport, running allows recreational athletes to compete against the world's best.

The only meaningful difference between you and people who run marathons in less than three hours is that they've been training a lot longer. Of course, there are gifted athletes who make any sport look effortless, who by virtue of the bodies and hearts nature gave them are capable of amazing feats of strength and endurance. In most cases, however,

....
SUMMARY
....

Too tired to exercise? Here are some tips for getting motivated.

> Exercise early in the day.

> Don't stay up late—turn off the tube and get your sleep.

> Reduce your intake of high-sugar foods.

> If you exercise after work, have a healthy late-afternoon snack to give you energy (e.g., a bagel, fruit or yogurt).

> Try different kinds of exercise until you find the ones you like best.

FACT

Morning is one of the best times to run, for several reasons. Not only are you statistically less likely to get hurt, but what you plan to do first in the day usually gets done.

their seemingly effortless performances are built upon tens of thousands of hours of hard work. And anybody can work hard, including you.

When you start to think of yourself as an athlete, you'll find it easier to be active. As most psychologists will tell you, imagining you are a certain somebody makes it a lot easier to be that somebody. You may be a recreational athlete rather than a world-class competitive athlete, but your goals and the efforts you put into achieving them differ only by degree, not kind. If you learn to respect those goals and think of the effort you put into achieving them as worthwhile, you will also increase your self-respect along the way.

Find your focus; the "fun" will come

Motivational experts will tell you that the best way to get in shape is to find something you have fun doing that also serves the goal of improving your fitness. When you first take up running, you may find the "fun" a little hard to discover. Although there is a lot to enjoy about running, fun is more a corollary than an intrinsic part of it. Some people seem to be naturally suited to running, and these people enjoy it immensely from the word go. If you're not one of them, focus on the reasons you came to running in the first place. If you wanted to improve your social life, think about all your new pals; if you sought the solitude of running, concentrate on that. If you came to improve your fitness level, think about how each step you take puts you that much closer to good health.

The really good news is that even though fun may not be the operative word when you begin to run, it certainly can be later on. By the time you have completed the 13-week RunWalk program and trained yourself to run continuously for 30 minutes or more, you will find yourself having more fun. You'll come to enjoy the feeling of robustness and power in your body when your heart starts pumping. You'll look forward to meeting up with your running partner or group for the social contact it gives you. Or perhaps you'll look forward to getting away by yourself and thinking your own thoughts as you pound through a forest somewhere at the edge of the world.

Seek out variety

Most beginning runners start off the program all fired up with an enthusiasm founded on a series of interlocking goals. As you move through the program, you will face increasing levels of physical and mental stress, which in itself can be highly motivating. Your ability to perform the tasks at each level will also provide satisfaction. But sometimes this isn't enough.

Dr. David Cox, a clinical psychologist who has worked with a large number of sports programs in Canada, recommends that you continually seek new ways to enjoy running after becoming involved in the sport. For example, you may find running around your neighborhood sufficiently rewarding in the beginning, but over time the experience may pale—you've seen the same garbage cans and been chased by the same dogs so many times that you don't think you can stand it any more. When this happens, it's time to change your running habits. Find a different place to run. Go exploring. Run in the park or along a beach. Go running in the country. Take your dog with you. Change the time of day that you run. There's no need to let running become stale.

Run with others

Another way to spark your enthusiasm is to run with a partner or group. Running with other people not only gives you a social occasion to look forward to but also makes you accountable: you are expected to appear. Joining a running group can pay off in many ways. People who join running groups are often as disparate as the creatures gathering around a jungle watering hole, but when it comes to running

....
SUMMARY
....

How to succeed in setting goals

> Set specific goals that can be measured.

> Resist the temptation to compare yourself with others.

> Set a deadline for achieving your goals.

> Set challenging but realistic goals.

> Set both short-term and long-term goals.

> Set positive rather than negative goals.

> Evaluate your progress and take time to congratulate yourself.

they are equals sharing a passion for a similar activity. Running is a great social equalizer: when you're moving down the road together, nobody cares if you're a brain surgeon or a janitor, a lawyer or a coffee-shop barista. You are a brother or sister in the cause, and just as the people you run with are the impetus for you overcoming your inertia, you get them going. Sometimes there are other payoffs as well, including social activities apart from running, such as brunches or dinner outings. You never know; you might even meet someone special. (Running groups are not a pick-up scene for singles, but it's not as though love has never blossomed somewhere between miles 6 and 7.)

Make running a time for you

Group running isn't for everyone. Some people find that being alone is what makes running worth all the effort. People who feel crowded between their work and home lives often resort to running because it's the only time they have to be alone with themselves. Sport psychologist David Cox believes that running after you leave work and before you arrive home at the end of the day could be one of the best things you can do for your sanity. "The literature suggests that most people who burn out need some kind of decompression between work and home, and exercise can operate as a great buffer between the two. Sometimes a run after work and before you start to interact with your family can have a really positive impact on your home life. It allows you to decompress in a safe way and is a lot healthier than going to a bar or going home and mixing a drink."

If you're bedeviled by stress, constantly worrying that your life is out of balance, a regular running program can give you an area of your life that you can truly call your own, one that you can control when everything else seems tinged with madness. That feeling of control may even wash over into the rest of your life.

With the emergence of social media, online networks are becoming an integral part of our personal and professional lives. The fact is, it is not always easy to find people who are as committed to learning to run as you are, and joining one of the many online running support groups might just provide you with the support you're looking for. There is also a wealth of great information to be found on the Internet (see Resources and References, pages 207–10), but don't use it to change your training program. Stick with the plan for the SportMed 13-week RunWalk program.

Keep track of your tracks

As mentioned in the previous chapter, keeping a training log can help to keep you motivated. Like running with friends, having a logbook sets up accountability: if you start out keeping notes in your logbook, you'll find it difficult to avoid your responsibilities because those blank logbook pages will be staring you in the face.

....
SUMMARY

No time to exercise?

> Go for a brisk walk on your lunch break.

> Get off the bus a few stops early and walk part of the way.

> Combine activities— read on an exercise bike; socialize by walking with friends; run on the treadmill while watching TV.

IT TOOK the birth of her second child when she was 37 to make Teresa think running was something she needed to incorporate into her life. "About four weeks after the birth of my second child, I looked in the mirror and didn't like what I saw," she recalls. Now, even though she has a busy career as a nurse and two children to raise, Teresa never has any problem finding the time to run. "There's always half an hour or an hour," she says. "You just have to make yourself get up and do it."

She has a couple of useful tricks to make it happen, too. First, she makes a point of scheduling her run into her day well in advance. "If I tell myself early in the day that's what I'm going to do, then I usually do it." The other trick is even more cagey. "If I don't feel like going, I just put on my running gear anyway. By the time I get it on, it just makes sense to get out there and do it."

....
RUNNER PROFILE

Teresa

Similarly, keeping a logbook can help you schedule your training sessions. Suppose that you've written "Training Session" in your appointment book for 4 p.m. Wednesday. If someone phones you to propose a meeting at 4:30 on Wednesday, you can tell them you already have something on then and suggest a different time. A firm date with yourself can give you the backbone to say "no" to events that would compromise your training.

Forgive yourself

Of course there will be days when life takes over and you won't be able to do your training. You may be five weeks into the program, making great progress and feeling really good about yourself. You may be beginning to lose a little weight and starting to notice the extra energy that comes with getting fitter. Then something happens to interrupt your training. Maybe you go on a vacation, or you are under a lot of pressure at work. The bottom line is that you just can't find the time to run. Because you miss a couple of weeks, you may assume that you're back to square one.

ALTHOUGH he'd always thought about running, by the time he turned 60 and retired from his job, he was ready. "Deep down in my heart I always thought of doing it to see if I could." His wife heard about the 13-week RunWalk program, and Raymond decided to give it a try. "It was very difficult for me at the start, and there were times I didn't think I was going to be able to finish," he says.

Raymond points out two things that made him complete the program and run in a 10-k race. "One, I'm the kind of person who goes all out, so without the regimented program I possibly would have tried to run too far too soon and ended up thinking running wasn't for me." And the second thing? "There were times I thought about quitting, but my wife wouldn't let me!"

This is not the time to lose heart. For one thing, your body is probably in better shape than you believe. Once you have gotten in shape, it takes a shorter period of time to achieve that same level of fitness again.

Even if the worst happens—you quit and have to go back to the beginning of the 13-week program and start all over—so what? People often try to stop smoking several times before they succeed; that doesn't make either the goal or the final achievement any less worthy. You may be encouraged to know that elite athletes often use a plan similar to the 13-week RunWalk program to get back in shape after a serious injury. If starting back at the beginning works for them, it can work for you.

Talk to yourself—the right way

Most athletes have found that there are few opponents as formidable as their own psyche. Sport is a process of making mistakes; what matters is that participants are able to rise above their mistakes and respect themselves enough to come back and do better the next time. As sport psychologist David Cox points out, negative self-talk tends to beget negative results. The next time you find yourself engaging in negative self-talk, ask yourself whether it has ever made you any better at what you were trying to do. If you have trouble following your training schedule, instead of berating yourself for failing, try insisting on believing that you will complete the 13-week RunWalk program.

Use your warm-up for motivation

If you feel dozy after a long day at work, warming up can be invaluable. In addition to preparing your body for exercise and preventing injuries, a warm-up can get you going psychologically, moving more oxygenated blood through your unwilling brain and spurring you on. If you really don't want to run, persuade yourself to do your warm-up anyway. By the time you're finished, you may well feel like running.

....
SUMMARY
....
Stress-busting tips
> Exercise regularly.
> Eat sensibly.
> Get adequate sleep.
> Don't sweat the small stuff.
> Visualize something positive to calm yourself.
> Learn to say "no."
> Set priorities.
> Keep your cool.
> Do your best and leave the rest.

If you do manage to push yourself into doing your training when you just don't feel like it—as opposed to when your body is calling out for a necessary break (see "Listen to Your Body," on page 61)—over time you'll begin to feel good about being able to take on apathy and inertia and win. These kinds of victories feed on themselves. The more times you win, the more times you will think you can win, and the more times you think you can win, the more times you will win.

Remind yourself that it will get easier

The farther you go in the training process, the easier it gets. For the first three or four months of your new athletic life, running will probably be a conscious event for your mind, just as it will be for your heart, lungs, knees and ankles. As Dr. Tim Noakes puts it, "The difficult thing is to get through that initial phase where you're thinking about your feet or your breathing or how you're never going to get through another lap and if you do it will probably kill you." But after those first months, running becomes an unconscious activity, he says, and "eventually, as the mind takes over, you stop thinking about these things. Given time, the mind will become as developed as the cardiovascular system and the musculoskeletal system."

Not only does it become easier mentally, but if you stick to the program and avoid the temptation to jump ahead, you'll go from one training level to the next with about as little physical strain as is possible in any fitness endeavor.

Hold a mental dress rehearsal

Mental rehearsal is all about imagining yourself engaged in the activity you want to have control over, as a way of preparing your mind and body for doing it.

Think about what happens when you're asleep. No doubt at some point in your life you've had a dream so vivid that it shook you into a physical response, perhaps even one so strong that it woke you up. Caught up in the passion of the moment, your mind was unable to separate dream from reality, and so powerful was the impulse to move that you leaped into consciousness. That same power of the mind to spur your body to action can be available to you during your waking hours. As an experiment, try to imagine yourself on your favorite running route. Start at the beginning and feel your heart rate increase and the air flowing in and out of your lungs. Imagine that you feel strong and alive and that if you wanted to, you could veer off course and run up the nearest mountain with relative ease. Now, doesn't that make you feel like running?

BREAK THE BARRIERS

Life is hard; excuses are easy. Here are a few common barriers to exercise and some practical ways to overcome them.

> You're a hard-working mother and you don't want to cheat your family by taking time out for exercise... Remind yourself that a healthy, happy mother with a positive sense of self will have more energy and patience for her family.

> You hate the way you look and you don't want other people to see your body... Try wearing functional clothing that you feel comfortable in and perhaps even do your running somewhere private. In time you will feel better about yourself, when you begin to feel more comfortable with the exercise program.

> You work a full day in the office, you have social and family obligations on top of that, and you're too darn tired to run... Lethargy breeds lethargy. It may seem contradictory, but to get energy you have to spend energy. The more you do, the more you will be able to do.

> It's raining. It's too cold. It's too hot... Dress for the weather and get out there.

CHAPTER 5 SUMMARY

....

1. Focus on your training, but listen to your body and consider taking a break if you are sick or injured.
2. Stay motivated by thinking of yourself as an athlete, seeking out variety, running with others and making running a time for you.
3. Forgive yourself if you miss a workout or have a bad run, and remember that even the best runners have off days.
4. Stay positive by focusing on the gains you are making, the goals you are striving toward and the good feelings that come with exercise.

6

The Family that Runs Together

....

CHILDREN LEARN about diet and exercise from their parents. Studies show that families that play together and make exercise a regular part of their lives are much more likely to have children who view exercise as an everyday practice. Regardless of whether you walk for half an hour to the park with your seven-year-old or run with your dog and baby jogger, the point is you are outside, away from the television set—and active.

We all know that a sedentary lifestyle isn't good for us. But as many of us also know firsthand, finding the time and motivation to get active—and stay active—is not always easy. The demands of work, family and pregnancy can make it very difficult to stick with any sort of fitness program. From pregnancy and purchasing a jogging stroller to teaching your puppy to run with you, this chapter will give you the facts on family fitness and strategies for staying active as your family grows.

RUNNING WHILE PREGNANT

You don't have to look far to see pregnant women exercising. They are everywhere: stretching in yoga classes, lifting weights at the

SUMMARY

Expecting moms
exercise to

> improve energy levels
> fight postnatal
  depression
> prepare for the stress of
  delivery
> improve sleep
> reduce the chance of
  gestational diabetes
  and pregnancy-induced
  hypertension
> maintain healthy
  weight gain
> help oxygenate the
  blood (which improves
  energy levels)
> promote muscle tone
  (which helps in the
  delivery process)
> reduce common com-
  plaints such as leg
  cramps and constipation
> lower blood pressure

local health club and jogging the trails and streets of every community. However, many women continue to ask if it's okay to run and exercise while pregnant. The short answer is yes. According to Dr. Karen Nordahl, physician and co-author of *Fit to Deliver: Prenatal Fitness Program*, "A woman can run as long as she feels comfortable and has no pregnancy or orthopedic complications. In fact, women who were regular runners before becoming pregnant usually find they can run long into their pregnancy, and for some, right up until delivery."

If you weren't a runner before you became pregnant, however, now is not the time to start running. Instead, try walking, stretching or taking a prenatal exercise class at your local community center.

In Dr. Nordahl's *Fit to Deliver*, she discusses the importance of a prenatal fitness program for both mom and baby. According to Nordahl's studies, a fitness regimen for expecting moms usually translates into strong, healthy mothers who have more comfortable pregnancies and an easier time in the delivery room than their more sedentary counterparts. The benefits are far-reaching, from reduced rates of pregnancy-related diabetes and high blood pressure to fewer c-section deliveries and shorter labors. Furthermore, tests show that infants born to exercising moms develop motor and language skills earlier—and more effectively—than their playmates.

Nutrition tips for pre- and postnatal women

Registered sport dietitian Patricia Chuey says that "overall, the recommendations for healthy eating for the general public are the same for pregnant or lactating women." Here are some of her suggestions:

> Emphasize whole grains and cereals, plenty of brightly colored fruits and vegetables, low-fat milk or milk alternatives and lean meats, fish, poultry or other protein sources.
> Consume three to four servings of dairy or other fortified dairy alternatives per day (one serving = one glass of milk or

other fortified beverage, ¾ cup/150 mL yogurt or ¾ oz/50 g cheese).

> Daily, choose good dietary sources of iron: meat, poultry, fish, cream of wheat, enriched breads and cereals, fortified tofu, white and kidney beans, spinach and oysters.
> Eat a meal or snack every two to three hours.
> Select snack foods that fit into one of the four food groups.
> Drink at least six glasses of fluids, including water, per day. (You want to have urine that is pale in color.) Proper hydration is especially important for exercising women during pregnancy and while breast-feeding, to ensure that milk supply is maintained.
> During the first trimester, women who are not exercising should consume approximately 100 additional calories per day (the equivalent of one extra snack). During the second and third trimesters, women need an additional 300 calories per day (the equivalent of two additional snacks or slightly larger portions at meals). If a woman is running, she will need to take in even more calories, depending on exercise duration and exertion level.
> Listen to your body and allow your appetite to guide your food intake. This means making healthy food choices as often as possible and listening to internal hunger cues. (Avoid being influenced by external stimuli, such as social pressure.)

Words of caution for pregnant runners

While most women are able to exercise regularly with few problems while pregnant, it's still important to run smart:

> If you are a non-runner who is now pregnant, this is not the time to take up running. Instead, try other activities such as walking, swimming or prenatal yoga classes—discussed later in this chapter. These options will be less of a shock to your changing body.
> Monitor any pelvic or abdominal discomfort. If you experience such pains or if you are spotting after running or high-impact activities, speak with your doctor as soon as possible.

> If running is too uncomfortable, try walking, swimming or pool running. These are great activities that put less stress on the body and joints yet still provide the benefits of exercise.
> Use common sense: avoid exercising in environments that are overly hot or humid, and avoid even mild dehydration.
> Make sure you're not working too hard, by using the talk test. If you find it difficult to speak, you are pushing yourself too much. If this is the case, stop and take a break until your breathing rate is normal again and you can easily converse.
> Physicians no longer suggest that pregnant women check for maximum pulse rates during exercise. There is no evidence that it is necessary to restrict exercise when your pulse rate reaches some predetermined level.
> During the later stages of pregnancy, most women feel a "shift" in their center of gravity. This means your balance is reduced. If you find running uncomfortable at this point, it's time to stop and try something else. If you are able to run up until delivery, avoid bumpy terrain and stick to flat surfaces.

Besides running, what can I do to stay fit?

As physiotherapist Denise Morbey says, "It's important for all expecting mothers to listen to their bodies." For some women, regardless of fitness level, running during pregnancy is just too uncomfortable. For others, their doctors have advised against it for health reasons. But don't become frustrated. Think of this as a time to try new activities. Cross training can help maintain total body fitness until you resume your regular running routine. Remember, this isn't the time to be concerned with improving your fitness. Staying active and healthy are better goals. Here are some ideas:

Swimming
> provides a great non-impact workout
> assists in maintaining aerobic fitness, upper body strength, muscle endurance and breath control

Yoga

> maintains energy, strength and flexibility
> uses static stretches, movement, breathing and relaxation techniques
> ensures a variety of workouts through the many types of classes available
> provides support and networking by having fellow participants and an instructor in a class environment

Lifestyle activities Everyday activities can also increase your energy level, and short bouts of daily activity may fit more easily into a busy schedule than some cross-training activities. Here are a few examples:

RUNNER PROFILE

Jen

JEN is 35 and the mother of two. She attends regular yoga classes, runs a couple of times a week and walks a lot with her young children, both of whom were c-section deliveries. However, she found it difficult to return to her usual active lifestyle after her first c-section. "My doctor suggested it would take six weeks before I would be able to resume any kind of exercise program but, for me, it took much longer."

For Jen, the first few weeks after the c-section she was in bed most of the time; stairs and strenuous walking were prohibited. After six weeks, Jen was moving around comfortably. If she had wanted to, she could have started some light jogging, but she waited a few months before going back to her regular yoga class. "Yoga was a great activity for me after my c-section. Physically I was ready to exercise, but psychologically I felt vulnerable."

Jen is now expecting her third child and another c-section delivery. She's staying fit with a bit of yoga, walking and some light jogging. Her plan is to return to yoga sooner than after her previous deliveries because, in retrospect, she believes the classes helped with her overall recovery.

> gardening, raking leaves and mowing the lawn
> housework, such as cleaning, vacuuming, dusting and dishwashing
> using the stairs and walking whenever possible rather than taking elevators, escalators and moving sidewalks
> walking during lunch breaks at work

CLOTHING FOR PREGNANT AND NURSING RUNNERS

Pregnant women today have a great selection of maternity clothing and exercise gear to choose from, including running tights, shorts and tops designed to accommodate a changing body. Phil Moore, owner of Vancouver's LadySport running store, says, "Many pregnant women are now wearing tights that are cut in such a way that they sit below the belly. Some women simply wear a low-rise fold-over waistband tight, which is then useful after the pregnancy. My customers often find the newer designs to be more comfortable and fashionable than the traditional panel pants for the expanding waistline." He also notes that though the more conservative maternity styles are still available in most stores, Danskin, Moving Comfort, InSport and Brooks all provide maternity clothes that both feel and look great.

Even so, if you ask any nursing mother who runs, finding a sports bra that provides comfort and function while minimizing movement can still be a challenge. Some women find that because of the extra sensitivity and density of their breasts, they prefer a bra that eliminates all or most movement in the breast area. Some women find wearing two bras helpful. But at least there are many choices out there. Most bra and sportswear manufacturers design an array of exercise bras to meet the needs of all women, regardless of shape and size. "There are bras built into tank tops now that are sporty and modified for feeding," says Moore. Nike and Champion Sports Bras, for example, offer good choices. They also use synthetic moisture-wicking fibers so that women stay dry and warmer in winter and cooler in the summer."

The right running shoe is an equally important piece of exercise gear for pregnant and nursing moms. Given that your weight will increase and your balance decrease, it's essential to purchase a pair of shoes that meets your changing needs. (Keep in mind that when your weight increases, so does your shoe size. Your feet may "spread" and your arches fall.) All running shoe manufacturers make shoes especially designed for the female foot, and many of these designs come in various widths to meet the needs of the thinnest and widest feet. Ask at your local running store for advice on the shoes that will best meet your needs.

Commonly asked prenatal and postnatal questions

Q *What do I do about my increasing breast size?*

A According to physiotherapist Denise Morbey, "Breast size increases during pregnancy and even more so afterward, when breast-feeding." Morbey recommends that pregnant runners wear proper-fitting sports bras and notes that those with a T-back shoulder strap increase directional support.

Q *My feet are growing. Why is this happening?*

A Increased weight means increased stress on the feet, so pregnant women need to pay attention to footwear. Shoes tend to break down sooner, so it's important to replace old runners. If you're unsure about the support your shoes are providing, check with a footwear specialist at your local running store.

Q *My balance is terrible now that I'm pregnant. What can I do to improve this?*

A "With increased weight gain in the abdomen," says Dr. Karen Nordahl, "a woman's center of gravity shifts. But although balance is more of a concern, it's not necessarily a limitation for runners." One suggestion is to try balance training: yoga, or just standing on one leg and alternating, are just two of the ways you can do this. As well, avoid trails with rocks and roots in order to minimize the risk of falling.

Q *I'm pregnant and concerned about running because of the loosening of soft tissues. What should I do?*

A Soft tissues loosen with pregnancy, though as Dr. Nordahl points out, "running helps maintain a strong pelvic floor and stabilizers." Still, it's important for pregnant runners to be aware of their bodies. "Women should stop running if they experience any pelvic pain when standing or landing on one leg." If you don't stop, says Nordahl, "this can cause shearing of the sacroiliac joint." Pain may also occur in the belly due to the ligaments being overstressed during the impact of running. And soreness in the knees, hip joints, low back and feet should not be ignored. If you are suffering from any of these problems, consult your physician and discuss eliminating the stress of running on land in favor of pool running.

Q *I had an episiotomy and want to return to running. What should I do?*

A "The scar from an episiotomy, like any soft-tissue scar," says Morbey, "requires appropriate time to heal." She recommends waiting at least eight weeks before resuming a running program, though this can vary depending on the individual. More time may be needed if there has been an infection or if the healing rate is slow. Once healed, the episiotomy scar should not be a hindrance while running.

Q *I had a c-section delivery. Will this affect my return to running?*

A According to Dr. Nordahl, "A c-section will delay a woman's return to her running program. A cesarean section is considered major surgery, so it's important to give the body time to heal. The fatigue associated with caring for a newborn may also delay resumption of exercise."

AFTER THE BABY ARRIVES

Most women take prenatal classes during their first pregnancy to learn about what's ahead for them with respect to their delivery, but very few take a postpartum class to learn about things they should do to get their body back after having their baby and why this is so essential for their long-term health. After the baby arrives, women can usually resume running as soon as they feel able. Health care providers generally recommend waiting approximately two weeks after a vaginal birth and six to eight weeks after a cesarean delivery. Still, it's important to check with your health care provider before resuming your exercise program.

Diane Lee, a Canadian physiotherapist internationally known for her innovative clinical work on thoracic, lumbar and pelvic disability and pain, suggests that pregnancy and delivery increase the risk of both incontinence (urinary leakage) and back/pelvic pain because of the inevitable stretching of the abdominal wall and of the abdominal and pelvic floor muscles. While the soft tissue of the abdominal wall and pelvic floor will recover in time, some of the muscles remain lengthened and inefficient while others remain toned and tight. Occasionally, the abdominal muscles stay separated and prevent the core from stabilizing. For this reason, all women should be evaluated by a physiotherapist prior to returning to exercise/sport to ensure that all soft-tissue injuries sustained during delivery have healed, the abdominal wall has closed and the muscles are working appropriately and the pelvic floor is functional.

Before running, you may want to try some fast walking. Moms should be able to walk at a good pace for approximately one hour before attempting a run/walk program. The gradual and conservative approach to exercise found in the 13-week RunWalk program in Chapter 4 allows you to return slowly to running, with less of the impact time involved in continuous running.

As during pregnancy, it's particularly important for women to remain well hydrated, especially if they're breastfeeding. "If your vaginal flow increases substantially after your workout, you have overdone it and should reduce your

....
TIP
....

Tips for breast-feeding moms

> For maximum comfort while exercising, find a well-fitting, supportive sports bra.

> Be sure to breast-feed or leave expressed milk before going for a run, to lighten your breast tissue, make running more comfortable and ensure your baby will be full and happy during your run. (Some reports suggest that breast milk after running has increased levels of lactic acid, which may alter the taste. But many lactating moms say this is not a problem.)

> Take a water bottle and stay properly hydrated. Signs of dehydration include dark-colored urine and dry lips, mouth and skin.

> Be willing to alter your
  workout to run with your
  little one in a stroller or
  baby jogger.

> Ask your partner to ride
  a bike or run with you.

> Encourage your kids to
  in-line skate or ride a
  bike or scooter alongside
  you.

> Try a "destination" run
  to the nearest ice-cream
  shop; a picnic after your
  run together is another
  incentive for kids.

intensity by 10 percent for your next workout," says Dr. Karen Nordahl. You'll also find that your breast size has increased, especially if you are breast-feeding. Finding a good sports bra is key (page 78).

Kegels Named after the doctor who developed them, Kegels exercise the pelvic floor muscles that are attached to the pelvic bone—which act like a hammock to hold your pelvic organs in place. (To isolate these muscles, try stopping and starting your urine flow.) Dr. Nordahl and physiotherapist Denise Morbey suggest repeating 10 slow Kegel exercises throughout the day *after* urination (to avoid urinary retention and possible bladder infection).

Core exercises The core muscles of the body include those of the trunk and pelvis, which are responsible for maintaining posture. During pregnancy and delivery, your core muscles have tremendous demands placed on them. By strengthening these muscles, you will be better able to support your lower back and pelvic region once you return to running.

A strong core, or midsection, assists walkers and runners in maintaining proper technique. Core strength is not about having a visible six-pack or flat stomach—it's about strengthening your midsection. For best results, consult with a strength and conditioning specialist who can assist you in setting up a program that incorporates core exercises into your training.

CHOOSING THE RIGHT STROLLER

For many active parents, purchasing the appropriate baby jogger or stroller is key to maintaining or resuming their fitness regimens. Your child will use the stroller from infancy until he or she can walk a good distance, which is usually around three years of age. But with so many choices, how do you know which stroller to buy?

First, consider your needs:

> If you will mostly be walking with your child in an urban setting, it's important to choose a stroller that is easy to maneuver over curbs and down the narrow aisles of the grocery store. A lightweight stroller that is relatively inexpensive is likely your best choice.

> If you plan to run with your baby or take her/him on hikes over rough terrain, spending the extra money on a rugged jogging stroller may be a good option.

> Try out a few jogging strollers to find the one that's right for both you and your partner. Each stroller feels different. Some corner better than others, for example.

> Jogging strollers vary in height, length and seat size. If you or your partner is taller than average, your child will probably be above average in size. In this situation, you may want to choose a larger and longer stroller.

Essential features for jogging strollers

> a solid frame that does not collapse too easily but has an easy-to-use locking mechanism when fully opened
> wheels that are easy to maneuver in a straight line
> a handle that is at waist level or slightly below
> hand brakes that easily and effectively grip the tires
> a sturdy seat belt that wraps around your baby's waist and between his/her legs
> adjustable shoulder straps
> an adjustable canopy and, for rainy climates, a removable rain cover
> pockets or storage space for extra diapers, water bottles, snacks, etc.

When is it safe for a baby to go in a stroller?

Before placing a baby in a jogging stroller, most health care professionals recommend waiting until she/he develops some neck strength, which is usually at around six months. At first you can help support your child's head by running on pavement rather than trails. But you don't have to wait six months to take your baby for a leisurely walk.

Walking a few weeks after the birth of a baby is a great way to get fresh air and enjoy a change of scenery from a world that has likely been limited by diapers and feedings. Walking is also good for the health and well-being of your baby. As physiotherapist Denise Morbey says, "Children model what they see their parents doing, and it's never too early to start being good role models." You don't need to go out and train to run a 10-k race immediately following the birth of your child, but a regular walking or running program will help your youngster adopt healthy lifestyle habits.

Tips for running with baby

Wait until your baby is at least six months old before you run together. Babies need to be able to hold their head upright before they can endure the bouncing of a jogging stroller. Remember:

> It's okay to walk with your newborn to six-month-old in a stroller, but avoid rough terrain. Again, your baby does not have the strength to support his/her head and is susceptible to neck injuries.
> When first running or walking with a stroller, go easy and stick to a paved pathway or sidewalk with few bumps and turns. It takes some time to get the hang of pushing the extra weight.
> If you are new to running, try to find a short route in your neighborhood so that if you grow tired you can easily and quickly return home. If you have the energy, you can always do two loops!
> Make sure you bring extra water and a snack. Regardless of your fitness level, pushing a stroller is hard work.
> If you're a dad, or a mom who isn't nursing, think about bringing a bottle in case your baby becomes hungry while

you're out on your run. It can be a long—and loud—trip home with a crying baby.

> Run with a weather-appropriate cover for the stroller. Today, any good-quality jogging stroller comes with numerous covers that meet almost all weather conditions and that are easy to remove.

GUIDELINES FOR CHILDREN WHO WANT TO RUN

It is impractical to make general rules and guidelines regarding acceptable distances that children should run. This is because children grow and mature at different rates, making it next to impossible to lump them physiologically or skeletally into general groups between birth and adolescence. As a result, guidelines and rules for children wanting to train for road races, track-and-field and cross-country events need to be reasonable and based on the abilities of the individual child.

Lacey

LACEY is a 35-year-old scientist and a mother of two who ran for the first six months of both her pregnancies. "I'm not a fast runner, but it is something that I really enjoy doing a few times a week. Still, I found that once I hit the six-month mark, it was too awkward. I was concerned about tripping. And I was running so slowly that I might as well have been walking." Lacey made the decision to switch to speed walking and attend pre- and postnatal exercise classes at the local community center. She found these classes a great way to stay fit and meet other moms.

Lacey breast-fed both children for about 18 months. "My neighbor also runs, so we would take turns looking after each other's children while the other mom went for a run. And while breast-feeding, I made sure I fed my baby first." Because she exercised soon after both pregnancies, her children did not shy away from post-exercise breast milk. "Some mothers tell me their babies are fussy when breast-feeding, but I never found that to be the case."

SUMMARY

Is your child a runner?

> Make sure your child has appropriate running shoes.

> Ensure the running program is child-driven *not* parent-driven—kids need to have fun.

> Have your child run every other day; children should not run every day.

> Ensure your child drinks water every 10 to 15 minutes when exercising.

> Watch the temperature carefully: your child is more susceptible to extreme temperatures (both hot and cold) than you are and needs to be dressed appropriately.

> If your child complains of pain, visit a sport medicine practitioner.

As pediatrician Dr. Trent Smith says, "Expectations need to be flexible. It's also important to take into consideration the child's level of activity prior to commencing running. The more active a child is early on, the more they will be able to do at the start of a running program."

It is best to use common sense when planning a running program for pre-adolescents. The Canadian Paediatric Society says there are no clear running guidelines for this group of runners. Dr. Smith suggests that running a 10-k race may be too much for most children, but a Grade 5 or 6 student who has run a couple of 5-k races could likely run a 10-k race with some training.

How should kids train?

Children who want to complete a 5- or 10-k race need to train the same way adults do when they are attempting these goals. But to hold a child's interest, parents and teachers need to keep training fun. By making exercise play-driven, kids are more likely to be inspired and want to exercise every day. If kids see running only as hard work, it is unlikely they will want to exercise into their teen and adult lives.

Making running fun for kids

If your child expresses interest in joining you on a run or walk, encourage him/her to accompany you on a bike. After watching you run, your child may catch the running bug and want to run as well.

If this is the case, consider exploring local trails and modify the RunWalk program. Have your child run to specific landmarks along the trail, such as a log or a tree—then wait for mom or dad to catch up. Walk to another landmark before your child runs again. If you don't have easy access to trails, you can do this type of run around your neighborhood: your child can run to the end of the block, for example, or along the schoolyard fence. Always keep in mind that most kids don't enjoy running the same way adults do. By making it fun, such as participating in orienteering or geocaching activities that involve running, kids will see their time on the trails as a game rather than a training session.

RUNNING WITH THE FAMILY DOG

Dogs are one of the best motivators to get us off the couch and on the road to improved health and fitness. You'd be hard pressed to find more energetic and committed running partners. Fit dogs also have more energy, sleep better and are more aware of their surroundings than dogs with sedentary lifestyles.

Of course, like humans, all dogs are not created equal. Some breeds, or builds, are better suited for running than others. A good running dog has a medium build, weighs 50 to 70 pounds (22.5 to 31.5 kilograms) and has short to medium-short hair. Evidence suggests that retired greyhounds, Labradors, retrievers, setters, spaniels and working dogs such as border collies and huskies make good running dogs. Cross breeds can also make great running companions. Less suitable breeds for running include large dogs such as Great Danes as well as small dogs such as Chihuahuas, because of their short legs. Flat-faced dogs such as pugs and boxers also find running a challenge, because of their difficulty breathing.

Getting started

The general rule is that dog owners should wait until their dog is fully grown before running together. With smaller dogs, this means waiting until your pup is at least six months old; with larger dogs, you can begin when your dog is about one year old.

If you are a regular runner and plan to have your dog accompany you on most training runs, it's a good idea to have your pet checked by a vet to ensure there are no lung, heart or joint problems and that your dog is up to the challenge of a distance running program.

It may seem like dogs are made to run, because they are enthusiastic and rarely refuse an offer to run with their owner. But the repetitive pounding, pace and duration of a run can be difficult and harmful for some dogs. Running without stopping is unnatural for a dog. They are pack animals, with a natural tendency to push hard in order to keep up.

Most veterinarians and dog trainers suggest that dogs should not run longer than 3 miles (5 kilometers). A dog may display energy and enthusiasm to run great distances, but it is important to be cautious and conservative when planning the distance and duration of your runs when training with a pet.

Make a running plan for your pooch, even if it's a running breed. The plan should include a gradual buildup in time and

Suzy

SUZY is a 33-year-old single mother and teacher who loves to be active. She runs a few times a week and has participated in numerous triathlons. When deciding to have a child on her own, she knew that maintaining an active lifestyle was essential to her health and happiness. She was confident that running and walking could be done with a young baby.

A month after Lily was born, Suzy received a jogging stroller for her baby shower. She decided to wait until Lily was six months old before she did anything more rigorous than walking with her. At six months, she placed Lily in the stroller and set out for a 45-minute run. But she returned home feeling exhausted and disappointed. The stroller was heavy and difficult to maneuver, and Lily was fussy for most of the workout. Suzy was frustrated and wondered if the stroller was going to work for her.

A friend told Suzy that her expectations might be too high. She suggested Suzy's fitness level had likely decreased during pregnancy. Reluctantly, Suzy had to adjust her goals, but after a couple of days she found a flat course along the ocean that looked perfect. After a month of walk/jogging Suzy was able to run slowly for 30 minutes, and Lily had grown more comfortable being in the stroller.

distance over several weeks. This way, your dog's endurance will improve over time, limiting the aches and pains commonly associated with an overly aggressive schedule.

Some of the warning signs that a dog has done too much include increased saliva, vomiting, irregular breathing and an uneven gait. If you notice these signs, have your dog stop and take a break. If the symptoms persist, take your pet to the vet to be checked out.

It's important to be safe and aware when running with your dog. Training your dog to run on-leash is the first step. Make sure he or she stays by your side, to avoid running into traffic. If you are running on a trail, ensure you're in an area where dogs are allowed and keep an eye out for kids and bikes so your dog doesn't get distracted or have a collision. If you're running in the heat, be mindful that dogs do not get rid of heat the same way humans do. They pant and sweat through the pads of their feet and can quickly get overheated. Ensure that you are carrying snacks and water to keep them happy and hydrated!

CHAPTER 6 SUMMARY
....

1. Active parents who exercise with their kids are more likely to have kids who grow up to make exercise an everyday practice in their own lives.
2. As long as a woman is comfortable and has no complications, running during pregnancy—if it is not a new activity—is a great way to stay strong and healthy and prepare for delivery.
3. If running feels too difficult during or immediately after pregnancy, consider swimming, yoga or other lifestyle activities instead.
4. Core exercises and Kegels can help strengthen the abdominal and pelvic floor muscles that were weakened during pregnancy, making a return to exercise quicker and easier.
5. Make time to exercise as a family, by using a jogging stroller, having the kids bike or run alongside you and even including the family dog.

7

Becoming a
Better Runner

....

YOU'RE RUNNING, and you like it and would like to get even better at it. Near the end of this chapter, we offer some advice on improving your running technique. But there are a number of other things you can do to become a better athlete and improve your overall fitness, all of which will also make you a better runner. Among your options are cross training (which in itself offers many options), strength training and stretching.

CROSS TRAINING

Cross training means participating in a variety of training activities. Almost any activity that gets you huffing and puffing qualifies: skiing (both cross-country and downhill), cycling, swimming, in-line skating, ice skating, hiking, walking, climbing, circuit training and aerobic exercise to music are all excellent choices. By taking part in one of these activities in addition to running, you can increase your overall fitness and build strength in general instead of in areas specific only to running.

The benefits of cross training include resting certain muscle groups while using different ones. Cross training also helps athletes avoid boredom. The variety of different exercises can be a psychological boost.

Cross training will also reduce your risk of injury. Following the 13-week RunWalk program will give your body, from your heart to your Achilles tendons, the best possible chance to adjust to the stresses and strains of running. There would be no need for such a program if the stresses and strains weren't there. But running can be hard on your body, especially if you were born with some biomechanical imbalances (high arches, for instance, or a misaligned kneecap), or if you have ever been injured. Participating in other aerobic activities serves many of the same goals as running—producing good cardiovascular fitness in addition to increased strength, endurance and weight control—but shifts the stress around, so that it isn't all borne by the same parts of the body. With some sports—notably cycling, swimming, in-line skating and cross-country skiing—the musculoskeletal stress is quite low. Thus, by cross training, you'll get stronger, you'll be fitter and you'll also give your ankles, knees and hips a break from the pounding action of running.

Cross training strengthens the body and can actually make you a better runner than if you train just by running. Dr. Tim Noakes says that if he had his running career to do over, he would compete in more triathlons. "Marathons and ultra-marathons (50 miles/80 kilometers and up) are what really wear you out."

Cycling is one of the cross-training activities most commonly favored by runners. Cycling strengthens primarily your quadriceps (the big muscle group at the front of your upper leg), whereas running uses primarily the hamstrings (the big muscle group at the back of your upper leg). Developing balanced strength in "opposing" muscle combinations such as the quadriceps and hamstrings (see "Strength Training," page 187) is an important way to avoid injury.

Another activity runners often choose is cross-country skiing, because it's a huge aerobic challenge and works virtually every muscle in the body, both upper and lower. Of course, your opportunities to ski will be limited by the climate in which you live.

Pool running, which can be done in any climate, is gaining in popularity. Basically, you just jog in deep water while wearing a flotation device. Pool running is usually practiced only by the very dedicated and by people recovering from injuries.

Another advocate of cross training is Mark Spitz, the American swimmer who dominated men's swimming in 1972, bringing home a treasure trove of medals (seven of them gold) from that year's Summer Olympics. Spitz says the reason swimmers today are beating his times by very large margins is that they're not spending all their time in the pool; rather, they're cross training and strengthening their bodies in other ways. Similarly, at the recreational as well as the competitive level, cross training can actually make you a better, stronger runner than if you train just by running.

Another benefit of cross training is that in exploring its options, you may well discover another sport you really like. When you do, you can help your body adjust to its rigors by applying principles similar to those you learned in the 13-week RunWalk program.

If you are taking up exercise at least in part as a way of controlling your weight, you will want to know how other activities stack up against running in terms of energy requirements. The following list shows a variety of activities, from less to more strenuous. As the list indicates, running at a fast pace (7 minutes per mile/4.5 minutes per kilometer) is more effective in burning calories.

Finally, cross training helps you avoid the biggest enemy of all training programs: psychological burnout. It allows you to work at improving your fitness level without subjecting you to the same routine day after day, keeping you from getting bored.

··············
FACT
··············

Passive exercise devices—rolling machines, vibrating belts, vibrating tables and motor-driven bicycles and rowing machines—will not break up fat or help you shed weight. Massage will improve circulation and induce relaxation, but it will not change your shape.

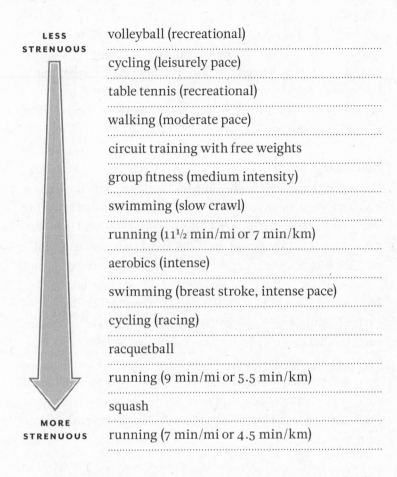

LESS STRENUOUS

volleyball (recreational)

cycling (leisurely pace)

table tennis (recreational)

walking (moderate pace)

circuit training with free weights

group fitness (medium intensity)

swimming (slow crawl)

running (11½ min/mi or 7 min/km)

aerobics (intense)

swimming (breast stroke, intense pace)

cycling (racing)

racquetball

running (9 min/mi or 5.5 min/km)

squash

MORE STRENUOUS

running (7 min/mi or 4.5 min/km)

In brief, cross training can

> distribute the load of training among various body parts,
  thereby reducing the risk of injury
> add variety to your workouts to keep you from losing interest
> allow you to continue training if you are injured, by using
  uninjured joints and muscles in a different activity
> develop your entire body, rather than only a few specific
  parts

More facts about some specific cross-training activities,
along with some of the reasons you might want to consider
incorporating them into your life, appear below. Keep in mind,

however, that you needn't limit yourself to just these activities. Table tennis isn't included, but besides being a lot of fun to play, it's a great game for working up a sweat and developing hand-eye coordination. No matter what activity you choose, remember to heed the three rules of training: moderation, consistency and rest.

Swimming

Swimming provides a non-impact workout, which makes it a superior choice if you are injured. It will assist in boosting your aerobic fitness, upper body strength, muscular endurance and breathing control. This last feature is especially valuable. Your muscles need a steady supply of oxygen, and although you don't want to breathe too deeply or too fast, because you can hyperventilate and make yourself dizzy, too little air will leave you breathless. Swimming teaches you to breathe rhythmically. It isn't very expensive and can be done year-round, both indoors and out.

It is important to keep in mind that swimming is not ideal for weight loss: water supports so much of the body that swimming doesn't burn as many calories per minute as running does.

Cycling

There used to be two types of road warriors in this world, those who ran and those who rode, but the benefits of cross training are making for a lot of crossover. Both groups are finding that the other sport complements their own and leads to a higher degree of overall fitness.

As mentioned in the general information on cross training, cycling enhances muscle balance between the hamstrings and the quadriceps, which can help prevent injuries on the weaker side. Cycling also provides a good workout for your legs with less pounding and jarring than running.

Cycling can be a lot of fun, too. You can cover vast distances with less effort and explore new neighborhoods and trails. Mountain bikes have an advantage over road bikes in that they allow you to get off roads you are forced to share with automobiles. Depending on how extreme you get, trail riding can be a very intense workout. Off-road riding doesn't require a costly top-of-the-line bike, just one strong enough to take the bumps.

On the downside, mountain bikes are ill suited to longer-distance riding and touring. As a result, many people are dusting off their old 10-speeds or purchasing good-quality road bikes.

Then again, you don't even have to go outside to go cycling. Some people actually prefer stationary bikes. Local gyms usually have a string of them; they are ridden by people who prefer reading magazines to dodging tree trunks in the forest. Stationary bikes can be ridden through all kinds of weather and can even be pushed in front of the TV set for those who want to combine fitness with entertainment.

Cross-country skiing

Cross-country skiing's big advantage over its downhill cousin is its low cost: not only is there no outlay for lift tickets, but the equipment you need can be less expensive, too.

Cross-country skiing provides an excellent cardio workout and, as with cycling, there's very little of the jarring and pounding associated with running. Cross-country skiing tests just about every muscle in your body—including the large muscles of your arms, shoulders, torso, back and legs—which makes it the ideal all-round workout.

If you're lucky enough to live in an area where cross-country skiing is an option, you will probably discover numerous skiers as dedicated and loyal to this sport as runners are to theirs.

Group fitness

Some men turn up their noses at aerobics to music because it has been deemed a feminine activity. It's their loss. Women do

FACT

There are no magic pills or special elixirs that can improve your running performance significantly. Improvement is accomplished only by training well and consistently.

make up the biggest chunk of participants, but these women can be very, very fit. They have discovered that pounding music, a group atmosphere and having someone calling out moves is highly motivating, and that the fitness results can be astounding. If you decide aerobics is for you, consider three factors to avoid injury. First, choose a low-impact class. The majority of aerobics classes are modeled along the step-program format, which is low-impact, so you shouldn't have much trouble finding one that's suitable. Second, make sure you won't be exercising on concrete. Third, check that the class is led by a qualified instructor.

Boot camps

Outdoor boot camp classes have been rapidly growing in popularity over the past five years. The majority of classes incorporate strength training and cardio in an outdoor environment, mostly using body weight exercises.

A word of caution on boot camp classes. Olympian Lynn Kanuka explains that you need to be careful before jumping into just any boot camp class: "Typically, in these classes, participants are asked to perform exercises quickly and aggressively. Many boot camp exercises involve a great deal of impact. While some boot camps are excellent, it really depends on the instructor."

True cross training engages the running and walking muscles in a way that does not involve much impact. Keep in mind that throughout the 13 weeks, you want to participate in activities that complement the running program. Running itself has enough impact, and an aggressive boot camp increases your potential for injury, which can have a negative impact on your training.

If you have been participating in boot camp classes before beginning your running program, consider decreasing the frequency of the classes until after you have completed the 13 weeks. Rather than two to three boot camp classes a week, try once a week to reduce the overall impact on your body.

In-line skating

In-line skating gets more popular every year as skates go down in price and up in quality. In-line skating can be done just about anywhere there are paved surfaces, which is a mixed blessing because blades and cars don't mix very well—all that sideways motion by skaters makes them a hazard, both for the cars and themselves. Provided you can find a safe place to do it, in-line skating will give you an excellent cardio workout and help build your muscular strength and endurance.

In-line skating is particularly good for strengthening the vastus medialis, the inside muscle of the quadriceps at the front of the upper leg, which is chronically underdeveloped in runners. Running develops the vastus lateralis, the outside muscle of the quad, so developing the vastus medialis will help you create balanced strength, to better support the knee joint.

Lynda

LYNDA, a 41-year-old office worker, "thought that running was one of the stupidest things on the face of the earth. How could anyone possibly enjoy it?"

After being diagnosed with a blood-pressure problem, however, she decided that some things in her life had to change. She heard that the 13-week RunWalk program was one way to ease into fitness and decided to try it. When she sprained her ankle (because of wearing poor shoes) halfway through the program, she temporarily changed over to cycling; later, she completed the program just in time to run an 8-k race in 50 minutes.

"On Tuesdays and Thursdays I ran for half an hour and then did weights. I'd go for light weights and lots of reps. I started doing it because I was told you can't improve your speed unless you improve your strength." Wednesdays Lynda alternated between finding a hill and doing speed drills. Her speed drill consisted of alternately running flat out for one minute and jogging for one minute—repeated five times. On Saturdays she ran with a group for 40 to 60 minutes, and on Sundays she did an endurance run.

In-line skating is low-impact—unless, of course, you fall. It's best to take some lessons and essential to wear the proper gear: wrist guards and a helmet are mandatory (a good bike helmet will do), and knee pads and elbow pads are strongly recommended. And stay off busy streets, because all the padding in the world won't help you if you collide with a car.

Climbing

Climbing is another sport on the grow, for sound reasons: it provides not only a good workout but numerous life lessons as well. Most people have a healthy fear of heights; assuming you're among them, when the going gets steep, you normally want to stay away from the cliff edge. In a climbing environment with ropes and harnesses, even though the safety system is extremely reliable, your mind responds to the danger. You're off the ground, if you fall you die, and it says, "Get back!" Of course, because you're there to climb, you don't "get back"; you keep going and you learn to work with fear. As self-help books have been telling us for years, groundless fear is what prevents many people from realizing their true potential, so sometimes pushing back the mental boundaries can be just as useful as pushing back the physical ones.

As a workout, climbing is good for developing muscular power and endurance as well, because you can be on the wall for a long time working out the moves. Climbers tend to have strong forearms, triceps, abdominals, back muscles, quadriceps, hamstrings, calves, ankles and feet. (A lot of that finger strength, by the way, comes from the forearm.) As with in-line skating, climbing is low-impact unless you fall. Although it's extremely rare for anyone to fall if the safety system is used correctly, climbing is still an inherently dangerous sport, so proper training is highly recommended. Most larger urban centers have indoor climbing facilities, and most of these offer training programs.

STRENGTH TRAINING

Some runners don't strength train because, they say, they lose speed if they bulk up. This is a myth. Strength training is vital to the development of speed. Although you can become a capable runner without working with weights, increasing muscle tone by strength training will help—and make running more enjoyable as well.

The main reason to strength train is that it can assist you in developing your muscles in a more balanced way, which reduces the risk of injury. Injuries tend to occur when muscle strength is insufficient to support weaknesses, whether those are naturally occurring or have been introduced by previous injuries. For example, if you sprained your ankle or twisted your knee when you were a teenager, there may be lingering scar tissue around these joints. By increasing the strength around these old injuries you can give the joints the support they need to keep the injuries from flaring up again.

Muscle groups are generally arranged in an opposing fashion and while one contracts, the other relaxes (in support of the movement). As a runner, you will be most concerned about the opposing groups that include the quadriceps-and-hamstring combination, the abdominal and lower back muscles and the calf and anterior shin muscles (those at the front of your leg below your knee). Some sample exercises are provided on pages 187–91.

As well as helping to prevent injury, strength training can help prevent the decrease in muscle mass that occurs with age (usually the result of reduced activity and the aging process itself), thereby lessening your susceptibility to osteoporosis and other diseases. Studies have shown that even the elderly can increase their muscle mass and enhance their bone density through strength training.

Finally, increasing your strength has a psychological benefit, too: feeling strong feels good. Although weight training and variations thereof that lead to increased muscle strength can be tedious in the beginning, in time it can be very satisfying to flex a muscle and feel the strength in it.

Cautions

Before embarking on any strength-training program, you should get instruction on technique from a qualified trainer, especially if you're using free weights.

Even if you do most of your strengthening with gym equipment, it's best not to rely on machines alone, as they tend to allow very specific, often limited ranges of motion. (The strength you develop will be focused in the ranges that you are working.) Free weights can provide more variety and a greater range of motion. Strength-training exercises have even been developed for working on large exercise balls. (See suggested strength-training exercises for runners on pages 187–91.)

Start with light weights and do a larger number of repetitions. As you become more skilled and/or wish to gain greater strength, you can decrease the number of repetitions and increase the weight.

No matter what your age or fitness level, give yourself 48 hours between strength-training sessions. Strength training can be hard on muscles and it is very likely that your muscles will feel sore for a day or two after your session. Part of this soreness is due to minute tears in the muscle caused by the exercise. Given sufficient time, the muscles will knit back together to be stronger and more efficient. But if you don't give your body enough time to recover, you can do yourself more harm than good. This is especially true when you begin; as you get stronger, you will find you can push your limits farther.

Although you may be developing muscles in order to run, this does not mean you should develop only the muscles in your lower body. Upper body strength is necessary for good running posture. For example, if your erector spine muscles (in your back) are weak, you will find it more difficult to stand up straight when you run and will tend to lean forward. This in turn will decrease your stride and your endurance.

One last warning: at some gyms, people hang around selling various drugs and supplements they promise will help you get stronger faster. Even if that's true, it's certainly a case of short-term gain for long-term pain. Drugs can do irreparable harm to your body.

Hill running

Why run hills? Maybe you live in a city such as San Francisco or Vancouver, where it is hard to avoid them. Maybe you want to improve your running fitness so that you can run longer and faster. Whatever your reasons, running hills can be both rewarding and tough.

Running hills works your body both aerobically and anaerobically during the same session. As with lifting weights, this

Darren

DARREN loved running and wanted to be strong, but hated lifting weights. "It's so boring," says the 34-year-old police officer. "But you have to be strong because in this job you never know when you're going to have to do a little wrestling." Then one day he met a recruit with a vise-like grip who looked like he had been born in a gym. "I asked how many days a week he lifted and he said 'none.' I asked him what kinds of drugs he was using, and he laughed at me," Darren recalls. Darren's new friend turned out to be a rock climber, and the reason he was so strong was that he started climbing at the age of 10. "The guy was solid steel and he never lifted weights. At least not exactly. When he was climbing, he was lifting his own body weight all the time."

Darren started going to the local climbing gym, and after a course of instruction he bought his own harness and climbing shoes. "I'm stronger now than I've ever been in my life, and I never get bored—there's always something new to climb, and you're too busy figuring out the moves."

type of running is resistance training. As you build your muscle strength and endurance, your legs will get stronger and you won't tire as quickly. Over time, knowing that you can run up—and down—hills will bolster your confidence and give you a whole lot of new places to train.

When you first begin to run hills:

1. Pick one small, short hill to begin.
2. Begin slowly. Pay attention to what muscles your body is using as you climb.
3. Run a short distance to begin; one to two minutes is enough. If the hill is longer than this, take a walking break and then try to continue to the top.
4. When you get to the top, jog or walk slowly back down the hill.
5. Repeat the slow run up and walk down two to four times to begin.
6. Listen to your body; if your muscles are straining or you're having trouble breathing, slow down.
7. Once you can comfortably run up and down your chosen hill, you can challenge yourself by increasing the length or grade of the hill, the number of intervals (the number of times you run fast up and slowly down) or the speed of your run. Be careful not to do too much too far too fast. Also remember that running downhill places a lot of stress on your joints, so take it easy!

Training on hilly terrain

Whether you are walking or running, hills are always challenging. As you make the climb, remember the following:

> Lean slightly into the hill while hinging at the waist.
> Keep your core (stomach and back) strong.
> Focus a few feet in front of you, no more.
> Shorten your stride; use small quick steps.
> Land on the balls of your feet and lift your knees a little higher than normal.
> Keep your arms pumping.

> Be patient and before you know it, you will be going down the other side.
> Make sure you take it easy on the downhill as the stress on your body is much greater on all your joints, muscles and tendons than when traveling uphill.

STRETCHING

Chapter 3 discussed the need for warm-up and cool-down stretches, and sample exercises are provided on pages 182–86. A few points are worth mentioning again. Stretching can make you a better runner by increasing your flexibility. Don't forget to warm up gently first with some walking or on-the-spot jogging. Should you feel particularly tight, knead your muscles between your fingers to get the blood flowing. (If you have a running partner, you can massage each other's muscles when necessary.) Ease into your stretching routine and stick to light stretching before your workout, saving your deeper and longer stretching program for after your run. Stretch before and after every run.

YOGA

According to Yoga for Runners' expert Mike Dennison, "Yoga is a natural fit for runners. Running is a one-dimensional action that stresses the same muscle groups, tendons, ligaments and bones in almost exactly the same way hundreds, if not thousands, of times each time we run." Yoga is the perfect way to complement running, which will in turn make runners stronger and less injury prone.

Dennison provides some introductory tips for first-time yogis. First, don't expect quick results. Like any physical exercise, progress in yoga is gradual and incremental, with peaks, valleys and plateaus along the way. But that being said, even small improvements in flexibility can lead to huge changes in how the body feels and performs. Second, find a good teacher.

And what about the bewildering assortment of yoga styles and names? The way to tell what's right for you is by actually

SUMMARY

Yoga can benefit runners by

> increasing flexibility in areas that are overly tight

> strengthening leg muscles that are underutilized in running (inner quads, gluteals)

> strengthening muscles that are not used in running (upper body, core)

> improving lung capacity through deep breathing from the diaphragm

> improving mental clarity and focus

> reducing overall mental and physical stress

taking a class. Dennison recommends you practice once a week at a minimum. Don't forget, yoga is a supplemental activity that will fit around your training, so how often you practice will depend on how much time and energy you have after your regular running sessions.

RUNNING TECHNIQUE

Technique isn't likely to hold you back when you first start running, but the faster and farther you go, the more likely it is to affect your performance. Good running technique can often be judged both visually and from within; if the running feels smooth and efficient, it probably is.

A great way to get feedback on your running technique is to join a running group. Such groups usually include runners of varying abilities, some of whom should be able to help you improve your performance.

This section describes a few basic components of good form for both running and walking. It's not necessary to memorize the list. Instead, as you read it through, think about your own running style, one component at a time. Keep in mind that the most important thing you can do to improve your running technique is relax.

Positioning

Feet Your feet should point straight ahead and be positioned parallel to one another. When each foot strikes the ground, it should be directly underneath your hip.

Thighs When your left foot strikes the ground, your left thigh should accelerate backward while your right thigh moves forward (and vice versa).

Hips Your hips should be flexible, allowing for a longer, more efficient stride.

Torso Your torso should be erect, with your pelvis tucked in (neutral position). Visualize running tall.

Shoulders and arms Your arms should swing naturally, starting at the shoulder joint. Walkers should keep their arms slightly bent at the elbow, their wrists relaxed, whereas runners should bend their arms at the elbow and keep their hands cupped. Runners should also focus on keeping their shoulders square and driving their arms backward, which will create a rebound effect, sending the arms forward.

Common problems

Beginning runners especially will want to watch for these common problems.

Overstriding Overstriding occurs when, during an effort to increase stride length, the knee locks as you reach with the lead foot. The lead foot then lands in front of your center of gravity, causing jarring and braking. In this position, the knee is less able to absorb shock, and sooner or later pain results. To eliminate overstriding, be sure that with each stride your foot strikes the ground under your hip and with the knee slightly flexed.

Upper-body twisting Running and walking are generally linear activities. If you allow your upper body to twist too much, energy that should be used to direct the body forward is expended in wasted rotational motion. What's more, if your upper body twists, your arms and feet tend to follow and cross the midline. Not only is this style of running or walking inefficient; it also increases your chances of being injured. Concentrate on moving your arms through 90 degrees while keeping your body square.

High hands, hunched shoulders When fatigue sets in, your hands will tend to rise and your shoulders to hunch. This leads to increased tension in the muscles of the upper body and wastes energy. Your shoulders and hands need to stay relaxed and loose. To ensure they do, concentrate on your posture: head up and eyes focused ahead; shoulders square, pulled back and down; chest lifted and abdominal muscles contracted (pressed toward your spine); pelvis in a neutral position.

CHAPTER 7 SUMMARY

1. Cross training strengthens and balances the body, prevents psychological burnout and can help to prevent injury.
2. Swimming, cycling, cross-country skiing, in-line skating, climbing and group fitness classes are excellent cross-training activities for running.
3. Strength training can help redress running muscle imbalances in the quadriceps/hamstring, abdominals/lower back muscles and calf/anterior shin muscles.
4. Running hills is a great way to build strength and power so you can run longer and faster.
5. Good running technique involves standing tall, looking straight ahead, swinging your arms naturally and pushing off from your forefoot and landing on your midfoot.

8

Fueling the Body

....

A CAR won't go without the proper fuel in its tank, nor will your
body. No matter how much or how little you exercise, whether you
are trying to lose weight or put it on, you have to feed your body
healthfully to make it work well.

This is true for everyone, but especially for runners. Exercise can
be hard on the body—even the exercise in the 13-week RunWalk
program, which is designed to minimize that hardship. Ignore your
body's need for proper fuel and you will put yourself at increased
risk for fatigue, injury and disease. Pay attention to the care and
feeding of your body, and it will respond to the demands of exercise
by getting stronger. Not only will your training sessions be more
productive, but you will feel better during them. Your recovery
times will be shorter, too.

Patricia Chuey, a registered dietitian/nutritionist, is amazed
by how many people ignore their basic nutritional needs. "People
make so many mistakes when it comes to nutrition. It seems we've
been socialized into bad habits. If people take a break in their day,
they usually sit and have a coffee! Or they unwind after work by
drinking alcohol and eating salty snack food."

TIP

Don't deny yourself the
things you love to eat—
just be moderate.

Sue Crawford, a registered dietitian with a Ph.D. in kinesi-
ology, understands that it's sometimes hard for people to eat
nutritiously in today's busy world. "It takes a lot of thought to
get into the habit of eating properly," she says. "Inappropriate
foods are always the ones being pushed." But there are good
reasons to resist the stream of junk food coming at you. If you
don't provide your body with the nutrients it requires, the
consequences can range from being tired or getting sick (colds
and the flu) more often to getting heart disease or cancer.

HEALTHY EATING

The three keys to healthy eating are balance, variety and moderation. A fourth key can be added in these times of highly
processed "fast foods," namely that food be as close to natural
as possible.

Balance is about eating from all the main food categories,
including fruits, vegetables, grains, legumes (beans), meat
and milk products—with exceptions, of course, for those who
choose to follow a form of vegetarian diet. Remember that
no one food group can provide you with all the nutrients you
need. A steak with a few peas on the side is not a balanced
meal, nor is pasta every day for a month supplemented by the
occasional trip to the salad bar.

Variety means choosing a selection of foods from each
main group every day to ensure a healthy diet. No single food,
no matter how nutritious, should dominate your diet or even
your intake from one group. Oranges, for example, provide a
lot of vitamin c, but eating oranges to the exclusion of other
wonderful fruits such as apples, berries, melons and bananas—
each of which has different nutritional strengths—will not
result in optimum health.

Moderation ensures that you eat neither too much nor too
little. Dietitians suggest at least five servings of grain products
and five servings of fruits and vegetables every day. If milk
products are part of your diet, nutritionists suggest at least
three servings of them per day (three to four for adolescents

and pregnant or nursing women). As well, each person should eat two servings of meat or alternative sources of protein (e.g., tofu, baked beans) per day. So, what's a serving? The following would all constitute an average "serving": a slice of bread, a bowl of cereal, a banana, a potato, 1–1½ cups (200–300 mL) of cooked beans, two eggs or 3 ounces (85 grams) of meat—which is about the same size as a pack of playing cards. Vegetarians who eat eggs and dairy products (also known as ovo-lacto vegetarians) and those who eat only dairy products (called lacto vegetarians) must rely on fruits, vegetables, grains, beans, nuts and seeds for the nutrients provided by the meat group. Vegans, who eat neither eggs nor dairy products, rely on those same groups for the nutrients provided by the milk group as well as the meat group. For vegans, fortified soy products are especially rich, useful sources of nutrients.

"Natural foods" might conjure up images of health-food stores, but the phrase really just means foods that either are not processed or are processed as little as possible. Such foods tend to be better for you because they generally contain more nutrients and fewer artificial ingredients than foods that have been more heavily processed. For example, potatoes are better for you than potato chips, bread made from whole wheat flour is better than bread made from white flour and apples are better than apple juice. This is not to say that junk food must never again pass your lips, just that it should play a minor role in your diet.

LOW-CARBOHYDRATE DIETS

Never before have North Americans been this unhealthy and overweight. Today's fast-food, 24-hour culture has changed not only how we eat but how much. It's not surprising that low-carbohydrate diets that promise quick and easy solutions to their weight-loss woes have millions of North Americans eating little more than steak, bacon and cheese.

High-protein, low-carbohydrate diets first became popular in the 1970s and then again in the early part of the

21st century. These diets, which advocate eating large amounts of protein while discouraging the intake of carbohydrates, present people of all shapes and sizes with novel options to weight loss that are easy to follow. From the sedentary father who wants to lose 20 pounds (9 kilograms) and gain energy to the athlete looking for a leaner physique, a low-carb diet does, at least initially, produce weight loss.

The "science" behind low-carb diets

One of the less understood issues about low-carbohydrate diets is how they initially promote rapid weight loss. According to sport dietitian Patricia Chuey, "The body mainly stores carbohydrate in the liver and muscle tissue. For every gram of stored carbohydrate (glycogen), the body may store up to 0.1 ounces (3 grams) of water. When people stop eating carbohydrate-containing foods, they become glycogen depleted, which also results in body fluid losses." The result of this diuretic effect is rapid weight loss, but not of body fat. As well, according to Chuey, these diets induce a condition called ketosis, which suppresses appetite and leads to reduced caloric intake.

When carbohydrates are reintroduced into the diet, the body stores them together with water. Subsequently, dieters see an immediate weight gain and perceive this to be a gain in fat tissue, which is not the case—it is mostly water. This is how carbohydrates get a bad rap. It is critically important to understand that the body needs a constant supply of carbohydrates for everyday functioning of the brain and muscles as well as for purposeful exercise, such as running. The few extra pounds that result with the reintroduction of fruits, vegetables and whole grains supply a healthy dose of fuel and fluid that is vital to sport performance.

What is not widely known about low-carb diets

> A diet that's low in carbohydrates and high in protein often produces immediate weight loss but rarely results in a permanent reduction in weight.

> A large percentage of low-carb dieters find this diet regimen too restrictive to adopt for a lifetime.
> Protein and high-fat foods are rich and satiating, but dieters quickly become bored and begin to crave carbohydrates.
> Vegetarians typically have difficulty following a low-carb diet because their food choices become extremely limited.
> A low-carb diet is high in saturated fat. Many studies show that diets high in saturated fat pose significant health risks.
> Low-carbohydrate diets are short-term solutions to weight loss or weight control because they are not practical. Restricting the intake of carbohydrates eliminates many mixed meals (such as casseroles), limits easy-to-prepare meal options (such as sandwiches) and complicates eating away from home.

Running in a low-carb haze

Fats and protein are not "clean" sources of fuel; when exercisers are forced to use them as fuel sources they don't feel good. Studies show that the effects of a low-carb diet on athletes is far-reaching. It has been proven that these individuals fatigue earlier, have less coordination and experience more irritability than athletes eating a balanced diet. So what do dietitians suggest is a good diet for regular exercisers? Sport dietitian Patricia Chuey recommends "quality carbohydrate foods, including bananas and other fruits, vegetables, whole grains, decent energy bars, chocolate, milk and quality sport drinks. While shunned by low-carb dieters, these foods are easily converted into energy and sugar and are well-loved by athletes because they promote faster recovery." As Chuey notes, carbs are still the main source of energy for active people. Without carbs, runners and other athletes report low energy and reduced ability to perform.

THE IDEAL RUNNER'S DIET

Runners typically train on a daily basis. Subsequently, their food intake has a significant impact on their performance, recovery and overall health. No matter how many hours they put in on a weekly basis, their bodies require that they choose the right amount and types of foods at the appropriate times of day. To attain the maximum benefit from their running programs, runners must satisfy the nutritional demands placed upon their bodies by running.

Sport dietitian Patricia Chuey stresses that "the ideal runner's diet consists of large amounts of carbohydrate-rich foods, including whole-grain breads and high-fiber cereals as well as red, orange and deep-green fruits and vegetables. These foods provide runners with the fuel they need to complete their daily workouts, plus vitamins, minerals and antioxidants to aid in recovery."

Chuey also urges runners to regularly include high-quality protein foods such as meat, poultry, fish and tofu in their diets. These foods supply amino acids, iron and zinc for muscle repair, oxygen delivery and proper immune function. As female distance runners may be at a greater risk than their male counterparts of becoming iron deficient, it is particularly important that they incorporate protein into their diet on a daily basis. Calcium, which is involved in muscle contractions, nerve transmissions, carbohydrate metabolism and bone maintenance, is another important ingredient in the runner's diet. Besides dairy products, fortified soy products, juice beverages and dark-green leafy vegetables can supply this vital nutrient.

In addition to food, fluid is an essential component of running performance and overall health. The perfect runner's diet includes adequate fluid intake—before, during and after exercise—to ensure that the body's internal functions, such as nutrient delivery, temperature regulation and removal of wastes, are operating at optimal levels. This is particularly important when running in warm environments.

PLANNING MAKES PERFECT

Eating right takes planning. Although you don't have to become an expert on the nutritional values of food, you will find it easier to stay healthy if you understand the basic ingredients of a healthy diet and keep those ingredients in mind when you shop. If you're used to living on fast foods or depending on highly processed foods, it may take you a while to adjust.

Pre-packaged foods and instant meals are often designed to capitalize on food fads; they also usually sell taste and appearance rather than good nutrition. These convenience food products can be part of a nutritious and quickly prepared meal, but you will want to read labels carefully and avoid foods with ingredients that research has shown may be harmful. For instance, hydrogenated oils can contribute to heart disease, and preservatives called nitrites have been associated with some forms of cancer, so you'll want to avoid these.

Put simply, you eat food so that your body can extract from it the nutrients, including minerals and vitamins, it needs to survive. No matter what kind of diet you live on, whether you eat fresh foods or not, whether you knock back milk like a teenager or avoid it altogether, your cells are looking for some basic elements to do their job. The body uses carbohydrates, protein and fat from food to create fuel for itself.

Carbohydrates

Carbohydrates are a vital source of energy that fuels both your brain and your muscles. They are abundant in any food in the grain group, such as rice, pasta, bread and crackers; fruits and their juices; vegetables, and, to a lesser extent, milk products and legumes.

Carbohydrates are important, especially for athletes, because they can be rapidly converted into glucose—which is the scientific name for the simple sugar that circulates in your bloodstream. Unlike proteins and fat, carbohydrates break down quickly; some can serve almost immediately as fuel for your brain and muscles. As well, extra glucose can be stored in your muscles and liver as glycogen, which is the main source of fuel for muscle movement. Human beings have a

TIP

The following moderate portions of high-carbohydrate foods are good sources of energy for runners.

> ½ cup (125 mL) raisins
> 4 Fig Newtons
> 1 good-quality energy bar
> 1 small whole-grain bagel
> 1 cup (250 mL) grapes
> 1 medium banana
> 8 oz (250 mL) orange juice or chocolate milk

low capacity for storing glycogen, which is why you need to replace it constantly.

Perhaps you are wondering if it wouldn't be best to introduce sugar directly into your system, instead of eating forms of carbohydrates that have to be broken down first. There are good reasons why you shouldn't. The main one is that sugar is a nutritionally deficient fuel, supplying calories but none of the other things you need at the same time, such as vitamins, minerals, antioxidants and protein.

On balance, about 55 to 60 percent of your daily caloric intake should come from carbohydrates. The daily requirement

SARAH had been running for a few years and had always maintained a healthy weight. However, after two weeks at her folks' place over the winter holidays, the 27-year-old teacher found that her pants were suddenly much tighter. She was not happy about the 10 extra pounds she was carrying.

After listening to colleagues discussing their quick results, Sarah decided to give a low-carb diet a try. She lost several pounds in a couple of weeks; the only glitch was her lack of energy. Prior to the diet Sarah had no trouble finding the motivation to run three times a week; after, she was lucky if she ran once a week. Her energy was drastically reduced, and when she did walk or run she often felt light-headed and moody. She was also fantasizing about bagels, pasta and cookies!

After two weeks, Sarah had lost 8 pounds (3.6 kilograms) and started to reintroduce carbs into her diet. She gained a few pounds but her energy was almost back to normal. While her pants fit a bit better on the low-carb diet, Sarah didn't like how the diet altered her moods and energy. She now tries to limit refined and processed foods in favor of more nutritious alternatives such as beans, fruits and whole grains. And while she hasn't achieved her original weight loss goal, she feels healthier and has more energy for her active lifestyle.

for carbohydrate consumption is 0.14 to 0.18 ounces (4 to 5 grams) per 2.2 pounds (1 kilogram) of body weight. Having heard that carbohydrates are a power food, some athletes load up on them to the wrongful exclusion of other important nutrients. It is not uncommon for athletes to get 80 percent of their calories from carbohydrates. But going this route can deprive the body of other important nutrients.

Another health concern is that the majority of North Americans get most of their carbohydrate calories from foods like white pasta and bread, and not enough from fruits and vegetables. Ironically, many vegetarians fall into this camp. "Grain-atarian might be a better word to describe a lot of vegetarians I see," Chuey says. "They tend to be eating all kinds of rice and pasta and not enough fruits and vegetables. The thing with regular pasta is that it's really just white bread in the shape of noodles, unless it's whole-grain pasta. I'm always trying to get vegetarians to eat more vegetables. Eating different grains is a good idea, too." Although pasta seems to be the carb of choice for athletes, it's a good idea to add variety to your diet by including some of the other grains—for example, brown rice, quinoa and oatmeal. At the very least, use whole-grain pasta whenever possible.

Protein

Protein is another essential ingredient in a balanced diet; it should make up 15 to 20 percent of your caloric intake. Experts recommend a daily intake of 0.03 ounces (0.8 grams) of protein per 2.2 pounds (1 kilogram) of body weight. For a highly active person this can increase to as much as 0.05 ounces (1.5 grams) per 2.2 pounds per day.

Protein is a requirement for the normal growth and maintenance of every cell in the body. Chuey says people easily recognize why children, who are growing, need protein, but have more difficulty understanding its importance to adults. In fact, the muscle fibers and cells in each person's body are constantly breaking down, especially if one is subjected to stress, whether emotional or physical. The body needs to recover and rebuild, and in order to do that it needs protein. By and large, however, an athlete does not need more protein per unit of body weight than an inactive person does, and the average North American already eats more than enough protein. Excess protein—whether eaten as food or acquired through supplements—can be stored as fat and can, under some circumstances, cause dehydration.

Protein is found in greatest proportion in meat (including fish and shellfish), eggs, dairy products (including milk, cheese and yogurt) and all kinds of legumes (including lentils and beans). Chuey and other dietitians, not to mention vegetarians, rate soy products such as tofu and soy milk as being among the healthiest sources of protein. Many people avoid beans, complaining of gas, but that's circular logic because the body can't produce the enzymes needed to digest them unless it's regularly exposed to beans. If you eat more beans, you will eventually digest them more easily and your gas problems should decrease.

Fat

Although too much low-quality fat is bad for you, no fat at all is even worse. Of course, it's important to distinguish between healthy and unhealthy fats.

The healthiest fat sources include omega-3 fatty acids, which are critical nutrients; your body uses them to produce certain chemicals it needs to function. Omega-3 fatty acids are found in fish, shellfish, soy products, walnuts, canola oil, flax oil, wheat germ and green leafy vegetables. Monounsaturated fats are also healthy, because they help lower the levels of harmful cholesterol (LDL) and raise the level of the good kind (HDL). Monounsaturated fats are found in olives, olive oil, almonds, canola oil, peanuts and avocados. Much of the fat you eat should come from these types of sources.

Polyunsaturated fat, which is found in safflower, corn and

sunflower oils, is also healthy, but less so than the omega-3 or monounsaturated types.

Saturated fats, the kind found in red meat, whole-milk products (including many cheeses) and such plant sources as cocoa butter and palm oil, are best consumed in small amounts. Finally, it's a good idea to minimize your intake of fats that contain trans-fatty acids. These forms are rare in nature but can be found in highly processed products made from hydrogenated plant oils. Manufactured foods high in trans-fatty acids include some margarines and many fast foods, snack foods, commercially baked goods (cookies, muffins, cakes) and baking mixes.

If you're trying to lose weight, eliminating fat from your diet is exactly the wrong way to go. You need fat to burn as fuel. If you eliminate fat from your diet, your body interprets it as a starvation message and instead of throwing its fat reserves into the fire, it holds on to them for as long as it can. Avoiding all fats is not a long-term solution to weight loss.

VITAMINS AND MINERALS

Vitamins

Vitamins are metabolic catalysts that regulate chemical reactions within the body. If you eat a balanced diet and take in the right amount of calories, your need for vitamin supplements will probably be very low. If not, it's alright to supplement your diet with a balanced multivitamin and multimineral, but don't delude yourself into thinking that popping pills is in any way a substitute for good nutrition: it's for good reason they're called supplements, not replacements.

Vitamin A is found in milk products and vegetables; vitamin C in some fruits and vegetables; B vitamins (including thiamin, riboflavin, niacin, folacin, B_6 and B_{12}) in meat, whole grains, yeast, green leafy vegetables and soybeans; vitamin D in egg yolks, fish liver oils, fortified milk and soy milk products; vitamin E in wheat germ and whole-grain cereals, and vitamin K in many vegetables, especially green leafy ones.

The sources of B vitamins vary quite widely, so deserve extra attention. Vitamin B_1 (thiamin) is found in breads, cereals, nuts, pork and ham; vitamin B_2 (riboflavin) in milk, cheese, liver, breads and cereals, and vitamin B_3 (niacin) in meat, fish, poultry, breads, cereals and nuts.

The member of the B-vitamin family called folacin or folic acid, which is found in green leafy vegetables, wheat germ, beans and citrus products, is essential to cell division in the body. Because the need for folic acid therefore rises dramatically during pregnancy, all women of childbearing age should take a folic acid supplement; doing so has been proven to reduce the risk of some types of birth defects. The recommended supplemental dose for healthy adults is about 400 micrograms, doubling to 800 micrograms for pregnant women.

Vitamin B_{12} is vital not only to maintain the health of your nervous system but to form blood cells. B_{12} occurs naturally in all animal products (meat and dairy), but not in any plant products, which is why it is the most problematic nutrient for vegans. However, a number of food products are fortified with B_{12}, including fortified soy milk and breakfast cereals; simulated egg, meat and dairy products; some meal replacement formulas, and nutritional yeast grown on a vitamin B_{12}-enriched medium. Vitamin B_{12} supplements are also available.

Minerals

Like vitamins, minerals are vital to your body's processes. Some of the more important ones are calcium, magnesium, phosphorous, sodium, potassium and zinc.

Calcium is an important nutrient for bone health and strength—from childhood growth, throughout an athletic career and into old age. Women, especially, should be sure they take in enough calcium as they need to establish good bone density before the losses associated with menopause occur. Both sexes start losing bone mass after age 35, but because women have smaller bones to begin with, they're much more likely to suffer fractures. Complicating the issue for women is that at menopause estrogen levels decline, further speeding the loss of bone mass. Current recommendations call for about 1,000 milligrams of calcium per day for males and adult females through to age 50, and 1,500 milligrams per day for females over 50. It's also important to keep in mind that calcium alone does not make strong bones. It takes weight-bearing exercise, and, for women, normal estrogen levels, to build and keep them.

Like other nutrients, calcium is best obtained from food sources. Milk, for example, contains not only calcium but also a protein that encourages stomach acid secretions that aid calcium absorption. The lactose (a form of sugar) in milk also helps with absorption, as do vitamins C and D (the latter comes to us from sunshine and is usually added to milk). Other good sources of calcium include canned salmon, firm tofu (made with calcium), fortified soy milk, dark leafy vegetables, sesame seeds and figs. It's a good idea to aim for at least three to four servings of calcium and/or milk products per day. For a list of foods that are a good source of calcium, see page 120.

Note: If you're not getting enough calcium in your diet, you may want to consider taking a calcium supplement. Calcium citrate and calcium malate are generally the most easily absorbed; it's best to take these supplements with food. Keep in mind that no matter how you get your calcium, if you take in alcohol, caffeine, salt or too much protein, you'll lose more of the calcium you take in.

Potassium, another important mineral, is found in bananas, most fruits, and potatoes. Potassium helps your body to transmit nerve impulses and helps your muscles to contract.

Food	Portion size	mg of calcium
DAIRY PRODUCTS		
Milk (whole, 2%, 1% or skim)	1 cup (250 mL)	300
Yogurt, low fat, plain	3/4 cup (175 mL)	300
Cheese, Swiss	1 oz (30 g)	240
Cheese, brick or Cheddar	1 oz (30 g)	205
Processed cheese slices, Cheddar	1 oz (30 g)	170
Milk, evaporated whole	1/4 cup (60 mL)	165
Cottage cheese	1 cup (250 mL)	140
Ice cream	1/2 cup (125 mL)	85
FISH		
Sardines, canned, with bones	8 medium	370
Salmon, canned, with bones	3 oz (85 g)	190
PLANT FOODS		
Calcium-fortified soy or rice beverage	1 cup (250 mL)	300*
Blackstrap molasses	1 Tbsp (15 mL)	170
Bok choy, cooked	1 cup (250 mL)	150
Tofu, firm (made with calcium)	1/4 cup (60 mL)	125*
Whole sesame seeds	1 Tbsp (15 mL)	90
Tahini (sesame seed butter)	1 Tbsp (15 mL)	63
Orange	1 medium	55
Almond butter	1 Tbsp (15 mL)	43
Pinto beans or chickpeas	1/2 cup (125 mL)	40
Broccoli, cooked	1/2 cup (125 mL)	35
Tomatoes, canned	1/2 cup (125 mL)	35

* Varies with manufacturer. Be sure to check labels.
SOURCE: Dial-A-Dietitian Nutrition Information Society of B.C.

Iron is an essential component of hemoglobin, the blood protein that transports oxygen from the lungs to the working muscles. Iron deficiencies can lead to premature fatigue. Athletes who ignore their iron intake are at risk for iron-deficiency anemia, as are women in general, as they lose considerable amounts of iron through menstruation. It is unwise to self-diagnose fatigue as iron deficiency and then self-prescribe supplements, because although iron is vital to your body, too much is toxic and can interfere with the absorption of such minerals as zinc and copper. Consult your physician before taking any type of iron supplement.

Ideally, you should get your iron from food. Good sources include meat, liver, dried peas and beans, asparagus, leafy dark-green vegetables, dried fruits, whole grains, prune juice and iron-enriched breads and cereals. (Check labels to see that they say "iron enriched"; if they don't say the

Gayleen

LONG before Gayleen started running, she knew the ins and outs of good nutrition. She'd been brought up to believe in the benefits of fruits and vegetables, and she tended to avoid the bad fats by default: she just didn't like greasy foods. "I felt I was way ahead of the game and didn't need to pay too much attention to changing my eating habits when I started running," says the 49-year-old professor.

The issue that emerged for her wasn't too much what to eat and how much, but when. "I like to run when I get home from work in the afternoon. Some people told me I should eat something before I run and some said after." Gayleen tried snacking before her afternoon run but she always felt sluggish.

"Eventually I figured out what was right for me," she says. "Now I avoid eating before my run—except for lunch, of course. Instead I like to eat right after running. Sometimes my partner and I even pick a route so we can finish up someplace where we can eat a meal or snack."

Food	Portion size	mg of iron
PLANT SOURCES		
Bran cereal with raisins	1 cup (250 mL)	9
Tofu	1/2 cup (125 mL)	7*
Potato (with skin)	1 medium	2.75
Pinto beans or chickpeas	1/2 cup (125 mL)	2.25
Parsley	1/2 cup (125 mL)	2
Raisins	1/2 cup (125 mL)	2
Dried apricots	10 (whole)	2
Broccoli	1 cup (250 mL)	1.3
Bread, enriched	1 slice	1
ANIMAL SOURCES		
Clams	10 (medium-size)	10
Beef liver	3 oz (85 g)	7
Oysters	6	6
Beef	3 oz (85 g)	4
Turkey (dark meat)	4 oz (110 g)	2.6
Turkey (light meat)	4 oz (110 g)	1.5
Chicken breast	1	1
Chicken leg	1	1
Tuna	3 oz (85 g)	1
Salmon	3 oz (85 g)	0.7

* Varies with manufacturer. Be sure to check labels.
SOURCE: The Gerontology Research Centre, Simon Fraser University

products are enriched, they aren't.) Iron is hard to absorb, so even when it's in the food you eat, your body can't necessarily use it. This is particularly true of iron from plant sources. You can dramatically increase your iron absorption, however, by eating iron-rich foods with foods rich in vitamin C; consider having a big glass of orange juice with your morning cereal or toast. Other good sources of vitamin C include broccoli, potatoes, strawberries, tomatoes, cabbage and leafy dark-green vegetables. In addition, you can increase your iron intake simply by cooking with iron pots and pans, which is how people from other cultures who do not eat meat, or who eat very little of it, get much of their iron.

Absorption of iron can also be blocked by certain foods. Fiber, tannins in tea and coffee, and other chemicals naturally occurring in food can all inhibit iron absorption.

The recommended daily allowance for iron is 8 milligrams per day for men and postmenopausal women and 18 for teens and menstruating women. Pregnant women require 27 milligrams per day. See page 122 for a list of foods that are a good source of iron.

....
FACT
....

Although there may seem to be a lot of rules associated with healthy eating, the rules still leave room for personal choices. Provided you eat a balanced diet and get the vitamins, minerals and other nutrients your body needs, you can establish eating patterns that best complement your life and running schedule.

COUNTING CALORIES

Once you decide what to eat, the next step is to figure out how much. Depending on the amount and type of exercise you are doing, you may need to consume twice as many calories as you would if you were not exercising. If you want to maintain your present physique or build, you'll want to think about the "calories in, calories out" formula. Simply put, your physique will remain fairly constant if the number of calories you take in equals the number of calories you burn doing work. (Keep in mind that you are constantly burning calories. You are burning calories reading this book and you are burning them when you sleep—not too many and not too fast, but burning them just the same.) If you take in more calories than you burn, they'll go into storage, usually as body fat. Take in fewer and you'll lose body fat.

Unfortunately, this is not always a perfect equation. Frustrated dieters know that eating less doesn't necessarily result in the loss of fat. If your body feels it is being deprived of energy, it will go into starvation mode and, at least to a certain extent, resist fat loss. It does this for evolutionary reasons—essentially because it doesn't know how long it's going to be until you'll start eating properly again. (More on losing weight later.)

If you want to get really specific about calories, visit a registered dietitian. You can get a complete analysis of your current diet and a program that will help you not only figure out what to eat, but how to plan your meals so that going to the supermarket isn't an exercise in frustration and dread.

SNACKING

Snacking can be good for your diet, as long as you snack on the right things. Consider an apple rather than a candy bar, a glass of milk rather than a soda. Fresh fruit may seem to lack kick if you're accustomed to candy bars, but your taste buds can be retrained. Most people find that after a couple of weeks of changing such habits, natural foods seem wonderfully sweet and the sugary assault of artificial sources seems cloying. Sport energy bars should also be treated as a snack, not a meal, no matter what the manufacturers claim; they simply don't contain enough nutrients to qualify as a meal.

PRE-TRAINING NUTRITION

There are two reasons why you should eat before your training session. First, you want to have enough energy to do the work—gas in the tank. Second, when you're training you want to be thinking about training and how to get the most out of it, not about how hungry you are.

If you want to eat a full meal before your training session, make sure you give yourself enough time to digest it: three hours for a dinner-size meal and two hours for a smaller meal (compared with about an hour for a snack). Your body can do only so many large jobs at once, so if it's busy digesting a heavy meal it won't be very efficient at lifting heavy weights or running.

Pre-training meals help prevent low blood sugar (hypoglycemia) and its accompanying symptoms of fatigue, dizziness, blurred vision and indecisiveness, all of which can have you making the wrong choices even with something as benign as running. Ideally, your pre-training meal or snack should provide you with nutrients that are easily digested and help maintain the right fluid balance. It should include foods you are familiar with and enjoy eating, partly so you'll eat well and partly so your system won't have to tackle something it's not accustomed to—your body is trained by habit to digest certain foods, so the enzymes you produce to do the job are unique. Provided you give yourself enough time to digest it, your pre-training food can be anything from a traditional Thanksgiving dinner to tofu on rice, but the experts recommend you lean more toward the carbohydrate group because fat, protein and fiber all slow digestion.

Your training period is a good time to experiment with different eating habits to find what works for you. This is where a training log can be helpful: it can show you patterns of response based on eating habits.

Here are some pre-training food recommendations that have proven effective for many:
> cold cereal, skim milk and a banana
> hot cereal with brown sugar and applesauce
> pasta with tomato sauce and a glass of skim milk
> crackers, a little cheese and some fruit
> whole wheat bread with peanut butter, some fruit and a glass of skim milk
> low-fat yogurt, fresh fruit and graham wafers
> a liquid meal: blend a spoonful of low-fat yogurt, 1 cup (250 mL) of skim milk, a banana and 1 tsp (5 mL) of vanilla

JUST DRINK IT

For a runner, water can be even more important than food. The human body is 70 percent water, and it loses water all the time through perspiration, respiration (breathing) and excretion. Perspiration is the body's natural air conditioning system: when you heat up the mechanism through exercise, you start to sweat more. To maintain your fluid balance, you must drink enough to replace the water lost as sweat. Sometimes the loss is barely noticeable, and athletes can be shocked to discover they have run out of fluid. Skiers and people exercising in hot, dry climates are particularly vulnerable, as they often don't notice how much they are perspiring. Sometimes the signal is a stinging thirst that can't be allayed no matter how much water you consume. Have you ever had the experience of suddenly getting thirsty, yet though you drank and drank until the water welled up in your belly, the thirst wouldn't go away? That happens because the "air conditioner" has run out of water and it takes time for your body to get the water you drink into the system again. This is why it's crucial for you to start drinking water early on in your workout, *before* you get thirsty.

There are other less obvious reasons to replace water lost through perspiration. Water filters out toxins and helps the body digest food and turn it into a form that moves easily through the blood vessels. It also helps transmit electrical messages through the body.

So how much water do you need? Lots. If you're not getting any exercise, the experts recommend six to eight glasses each day. If you're exercising, your requirements go up. How much they go up depends on how hard you're working out, the temperature around you and the clothing or equipment you're wearing. As a rule, it's a good idea to start drinking water well before you start exercising. Drink at least two glasses about two hours before you exercise and then another one or two about 15 minutes before you start to work out. Drink up to another glass every 15 to 20 minutes while you are exercising.

Finally, don't stop when the training session ends: drink another one to three glasses within 10 to 20 minutes after you stop exercising.

Note that these are guidelines only; the commonly recommended amounts may not sufficiently hydrate some people. The only way to know if you are properly hydrated after intense exercise, especially when the weather is warm, is to weigh yourself before and after exercise, wearing the same clothes both times or, better yet, nothing at all. (If the sweat has soaked into your clothing, you'll get a false reading.) Weight lost during exercise represents water loss you did not replace during your workout.

Resist the urge to follow up your training session with alcohol. Although you'll often see athletes tilting a beer after a workout, mumbling something about having "earned it," alcohol is a diuretic and will only make your already thirsty body more dehydrated. (If you must have alcohol after your

RUNNER PROFILE

Chas

CHAS started to run for only one reason: he wanted to lose weight. The idea of taking up running came to him at his 10-year high-school reunion. "A girl I'd known looked at me like she didn't recognize me. I had to tell her my name, and when I did she looked amazed. 'You turned out to be pretty big,' she said. I felt terrible."

Chas started going to a local gym but found the stationary bikes and treadmills boring. When he complained, an attendant suggested he join a running group. It would help with motivation and be more exciting than running in one spot. Chas hoped for instant results, and not getting them was discouraging. "It took me a while to learn that if I wanted to lose weight, I would have to do more than just run." It took Chas some time to change his habits, but once he got his mind and diet in sync, the weight started to come off. "My weight is going down, and I am pretty confident I can keep it going that way—hopefully until the next reunion anyway."

training session, at least try to down a few glasses of water at the same time.)

Of course, water isn't the only source of fluid you have to rely on. Most things you drink during the day will help meet your requirements. Coffee, although hydrating, isn't the best. Like alcohol, it's a diuretic, and with excess cream and sugar, it can be pretty unhealthy. Fruit juices are okay, but avoid heavily sugared ones (and heavily sugared anything, for that matter) because too much sugar in your gut will draw water away from your muscles. When you run, this can cause further dehydration, leading to nausea, diarrhea and cramps.

Sport drinks are more than just marketing hype. Some of these drinks replace electrolytes such as salt and potassium; others provide the carbohydrates and sugars your body will crave in the middle of a long race. Some drinks will do both. These drinks may be useful for athletes competing in long-duration (more than two-hour-long), intense activities such as marathons or triathlons, or training for more than one and one-half hours. For short-duration exercise—the type of training you'll be doing in the 13-week RunWalk program—water will do just fine.

WEIGHT MANAGEMENT

Seasoned runners tend to have a rather lean and hungry look, which is perhaps one reason so many people turn to running as a form of weight control. Although it's not an overnight cure, or even a short-term cure, running can be a remarkably effective aid to weight control. That said, becoming a runner requires patience and dedication. A lot of people who want to lose weight will try running and when they don't quickly get the results they were aiming for, give up. The fact is, it usually takes six months before the physiological benefits associated with running become noticeable and about a year before a runner's body starts to look really different. Consider how long it took to put the weight on in the first place. Why should it take any less time to take it off?

It's also worth remembering that a regular running program will not lead to weight loss if you eat low-quality food for dinner every night. If you want to lose weight, you must stick to a balanced diet and get prolonged and regular aerobic exercise. There's no easy way, no machine, no pill.

If weight loss is your goal, try to remember that you were born with a certain type of body. Being rakishly thin may not be in your genes. Some people are thin by nature; others will never be thin, no matter how much exercise they do. This does not mean that those people can't shed excess poundage, but be realistic about how much weight you are going to be able to lose and from what part of your body the fat will be lost. That "spare tire" of body fat around your middle will be a lot easier to lose through exercise than will fat on your hips and thighs, because fat located around the hips and thighs is controlled by reproductive hormones rather than stress hormones and is more closely protected by the body.

If you've been sedentary, it's important to start with lower-intensity exercise and progressively build up to a moderate- to high-intensity level, which is what the 13-week program does. Once you have achieved a higher fitness level, however, running at lower speeds will no longer be the best way to burn fat or achieve fat loss. Working at moderate- to high-intensity levels in either one 40- to 60-minute session or a number of shorter sessions per training day will burn more total calories and ultimately more fat.

One last warning: beware of fad diets. Fad diets are invariably designed to capitalize on people's insecurities and to make money for their developers, not to improve the health of the people who follow them. This is not to say that all diets are to be mistrusted, just that there's no magic to good nutrition. If you use the tools of good nutrition, chances are you won't need to search for miracle cures.

If you want more detailed information about weight loss—or about diet, nutrition or menu planning—check out some of the useful sources listed at the back of this book.

....
T I P
....

Helpful hints for managing your weight

> No single weight-control prescription is ideal for everyone.

> Exercise at moderate intensity, three to four times each week, for 25–45 minutes.

> To increase the rate of fat loss, gradually increase the duration of your exercise.

> To increase muscle mass, try to include a strength-training session twice a week. (Muscle burns more calories even at rest than do other body tissues.)

> Wait at least six months before you assess physiological changes such as improved cardiovascular fitness and increased muscle strength.

> Allow six to nine months for your body's proportion of fat to decrease measurably as a result of exercise.

CHAPTER 8 SUMMARY

1. The three keys to healthy eating are balance, variety and moderation—and unprocessed foods.
2. The ideal runner's diet includes lots of carbohydrate-rich foods such as whole-grain cereals, fruits and vegetables as well as high-quality proteins such as meat, poultry, fish and tofu.
3. Be sure to include healthy omega-3 fatty acids and monounsaturated fats, such as those in fish oils, nuts, avocados and olives, in your diet.
4. Drinking enough fluid—before, during and after exercise—is as important as eating the right foods.
5. Proper weight management is a blend of healthy diet, regular exercise, patience and realistic goals.

9

Common Injuries and Recovery

....

INJURIES ARE not only painful, they're discouraging. If, after putting in countless hours building up your endurance, you get an injury that prevents you from running, you have to sit idly by and watch as the fitness level you worked so hard to attain slowly slips away. If running is your main outlet for managing stress, you may feel especially frustrated and angry, and may even be tempted to dull the pain of injury with painkillers and try to carry on. This is the time to remember that injuries ignored are injuries that can haunt you for a lifetime.

Although it's true the 13-week RunWalk program is designed to minimize your chances of suffering a running-related injury, you can still be sidelined—as a result of an accident, overzealous training or your own biomechanical weaknesses. To remain healthy, it's essential to understand the kinds of injuries runners are susceptible to and the treatments offering the best chance for a full and complete recovery.

TYPES OF INJURIES

There are two major categories of injuries that runners should think about, says Hugh Fisher, a family practitioner and Olympic gold

FACT

During a mile (1.61 kilometers) of running, your foot strikes the ground between 800 and 1,200 times (500 and 750 times per kilometer) with a force of up to four times your body weight. (The exact force depends on your speed and the length of your stride.)

and bronze medalist in kayaking/canoeing. Fisher has had his own litany of aches and pains over the years, and he's also seen plenty of sufferers struggling into his office.

The first category of injury is the acute kind, which can sneak up on anybody. Such injuries are usually "traumatic," the result of sudden and violent damage such as a torn ligament (sprain), laceration (cut), pulled muscle (sprain) or broken bone. Traumatic injuries are best treated as quickly as possible by a qualified sport medicine practitioner, especially if there's any bleeding, a good deal of swelling or pain that lasts more than an hour. You should also attend to an injury quickly if you find it so debilitating that you can't walk or make use of the injured body part, or if you heard, or hear, any unusual sounds—popping, cracking or tearing.

Runners' traumatic injuries are most often caused by falls, from tripping over roots, curbs and the like. Unfortunately, the most interesting places to run are to blame for the most accidents. Trail running is extremely popular, but the unevenness of the terrain and the looseness of the ground often result in falls. Trail runners need to keep their eyes on the surface beneath them if that surface is uneven and be extra cautious about footwear. Shoes that don't fit or that lack adequate support increase a runner's risk of taking a spill.

The second category of running injuries—by far the more common—is overuse, or chronic injury that results from overtraining. Sometimes chronic injuries can be traced back to poor technique, but this is rare in beginning runners, who run neither fast enough nor far enough for technique-related problems to develop (but see the advice on running technique in Chapter 7 if you want more information about this possibility). "Overuse injuries often show up in people who are extremely competitive by nature," says Fisher. "They train every day and never give their bodies a chance to rest. Muscle and joint injuries are common, but sickness can also result, because they are just generally run down."

Dr. Jim Macintyre, a sport physician in Salt Lake City, Utah, says many overuse injuries result either from incomplete rehabilitation of an old injury, or from individual anatomical variations that lead to injury when put under stress. These variations can include flat feet, high arches or an abnormally sized or positioned kneecap. The results are the same: when there's a weak link in the kinetic (moving) chain—some part that's out of alignment naturally or as the result of an injury—the body compensates for that weakness to keep the person going. This usually leads to a different, new injury. For Macintyre, the red flags go up when athletes come to him suffering from a cycle of injuries to one side of their body. First it's the right ankle, then the right knee, then perhaps the right hip.

"Think about it," urges Macintyre. "How many people come in with one knee sore versus both knees sore? The mantra is to say it's the shoes, lack of flexibility, poor training methods, bad running techniques and so on. But generally, people wear the same shoes on both feet and run the same number of steps with both legs—give or take one or two—so how can you blame the shoes when you have only one sore knee?"

It's not that the injury can't be the result of the wrong shoes, poor flexibility, unsound training methods or bad technique, but that often the knees, heels, ankles and other sensitive links in the kinetic chain are the victims, not the culprits—the source of the injury lies elsewhere. For this reason, Macintyre, along with many other practitioners, recommends that doctors look at the whole body, not only when it's lying supine on a plinth in the doctor's office, but when it's in motion as well. Macintyre likes to see his patients walking and even running on treadmills to see how their whole body moves and where the trouble they're experiencing might originate. "You have to look at the whole chain. You look at the foot, you look at the hip and you look at the pelvis. You watch them walk and you watch them run," Macintyre says.

Tracking down the source of an injury is a bit of a detective game, according to Macintyre. "As a health care professional, the question you have to ask yourself is: why did they get this pain, and why in one knee and not the other? The obvious answer is that there must be something intrinsically imbalanced about the patient's gait. One possibility is that they're running on a sloped road surface. One leg is forced into a shortened position while the other leg lengthens, forcing the foot to pronate excessively. The knee becomes the victim in the whole thing. It has had abnormal amounts of stress placed on it as a result of something somewhere else that's causing the abnormal gait. It could also be something as simple as a foot that's not moving properly, a hip that's tight or a pelvis that's out of place due to a problem with the sacroiliac joint."

For example, in a properly aligned body, the kneecap should track evenly over the foot in a straight line pointing in the direction you are traveling. If something—such as a misaligned hip—causes your knee to track in another direction,

Helen

HELEN, 49, was trying to increase her running endurance in preparation for a race when she got a surprise from an old enemy. "I dislocated my knee when I was in ballet," says the retired aerobics instructor, who now works as an office administrator. "When I tried to increase the time I spent running, it was too much." Her weakened knee could only take so much stress before it gave out and she developed patello-femoral syndrome (runner's knee).

Considering the severity of her injury, Helen cut out running and went to see a doctor. His rehabilitation program returned her to running in less than a month, but only for 10 minutes at a time. "He recommended a stretching and strengthening program, and I also got orthotics. He kept testing the knee to make sure it was holding out." In a few months Helen was back to running for 30 minutes at a stretch, but continued her stretching and strengthening program because she had set her sights on a half marathon.

your knee will eventually be injured, and you won't even think about it until enough damage has been done for the knee to send pain signals to your brain. To make matters worse, if you, your doctor or your physiotherapist doesn't figure out the root cause of the injury, the knee will be treated and you'll go back to running as soon as it feels better. Then, guess what? The knee will be injured again. "To tell someone they have a bad knee when they come to you with knee pain is simply not good enough. If all you're going to try to do is identify the symptoms, then you say, 'Okay, this is patello-femoral pain,' you get out your cookbook and it says 'ice it, take anti-inflammatories and do these exercises.' But all you're treating are the symptoms, not the cause of the problem."

Sometimes the pain migrates to a different part of your body—your ankle or your Achilles tendon. Why? During treatment you probably did exercises that strengthened the muscles around your bad knee, giving it a greater ability to compensate for the problem that could be originating in your hip. The flaw then migrates to the next weakest link in the chain, then the next and so on.

New injuries can also be caused by old injuries that haven't healed properly. An old ankle sprain, for example, might lock one foot into pronation while the other supinates (rolls outward). Macintyre says he's looked at thousands of people with one pronated foot and one supinated foot and at first thought it odd these people were born like that. "But the truth is, they weren't born like that. Somewhere along the way something happened to the ankle that changed the range of motion or flexibility. The alignment was thrown out of balance, and the rest of the links in the chain started to compensate. Before the person started running, they may never have noticed this. There wasn't enough stress being put on various parts of their body for them to break down, but the stresses associated with running revealed the inherent weaknesses."

Biomechanical problems are not an absolute guarantee that an injury will manifest itself. Everyone's body has some ability to compensate: sometimes your body parts are strong enough to compensate forever. If, however, you exceed your body's ability to compensate, injury is headed your way.

Sadly, some runners get into a cycle of injuries and eventually throw in the towel. "I used to run," you'll hear them say miserably, "but my [fill-in-the-blank] couldn't take it." Maybe it couldn't, but more likely, these runners didn't follow the right course of treatment. If you do get a running injury, know when you're out of your league, and if you don't see fairly rapid improvement from self-treatment, get help from a professional who understands sports injuries. Sport medicine is not a strict discipline the way cardiology or neurology is, but an increasing number of medical practitioners focus on sports-related injuries. These practitioners include orthopedic surgeons, family physicians (such as Hugh Fisher) and sport medicine specialists (such as Jim Macintyre). Other practitioners who may focus on sport-related injuries include podiatrists, chiropractors, physiotherapists, athletic therapists, athletic trainers and massage therapists. You want someone who will examine the entire chain of your moving parts, someone who can assess the body in motion and not just look at localized pain.

If you are told to rest the injured part and just wait for the pain to go away, you may want to seek a second opinion. If the cause of your pain isn't treated, chances are the pain will come back when you start running again. An experienced sport medicine practitioner can both give a diagnosis and prescribe a treatment regimen, which will probably include alternative activities and a program of strength and flexibility training. By and large, you will find that sport medicine is more "aggressive" than traditional medicine in its treatment plan.

RUNNER'S FIRST AID
If you are injured, you should seek medical attention. While you're waiting for help, however, you can get started on RICE.

The acronym RICE stands for Rest, Ice, Compression and Elevation. It's standard procedure; everybody does it because it works.

RICE is often used in conjunction with anti-inflammatory drugs such as acetylsalicylic acid/ASA (Aspirin) or ibuprofen (Advil or Motrin). These drugs can reduce swelling but should not be relied upon as a crutch to mask pain and allow you to "run through" injuries. Also, remember that ASA and ibuprofen can be hard on your stomach, so take them with food. Note that although acetaminophen (Tylenol) is easier on the stomach and an effective painkiller, it is not an anti-inflammatory and will not reduce swelling.

Rest

The reason for rest is straightforward: if you've damaged something, putting more stress on it can only make it worse. But taking things easy doesn't mean you have to spend three weeks on the couch watching TV before you can use the injured part. Complete immobility is rarely recommended, the possible exception being in acute traumatic cases, and even then doctors will try to get you up and moving as soon as possible.

Moving injured parts is important because it stimulates blood flow to the injured soft tissue. In fact, anything that stimulates blood flow will encourage healing, which is why so many physiotherapists use ultrasound and similar stimulation techniques. Most of the time, however, unless you get in the way, your body's own healing powers will regenerate and restore damaged soft tissue.

A sport medicine practitioner will often recommend certain exercises to go along with RICE. These are usually designed to strengthen the muscles around the injury in order to help your body compensate. By strengthening the muscles around a vital part, such as the knee, you can support that part and make it easier for it to do its job. Exercises can also be designed to increase flexibility and enhance circulation, thereby spurring on the natural healing process. So do your exercises; they will make it easier for you to withstand the stress of returning to your activity because you will be stronger and more flexible than when you were injured in the first place.

Ice

You've no doubt noticed that swelling occurs when you injure yourself. This swelling is actually part of the healing process. It may seem contradictory, but even though swelling is part of the healing process, too much of it slows healing. Applying ice causes what is known as vasoconstriction of the local blood vessels in the area surrounding the injury, which limits bleeding and thereby reduces swelling in the area.

By reducing swelling, icing reduces the recovery time, so the sooner you can ice an injury the better. Obviously you won't always have an ice pack with you when you run, but in an emergency, cold water will help immensely. If you're desperate, use the water from your water bottle to soak your T-shirt and wrap the injury. If you can, hold the injured part under cold water until you can find some ice and properly apply it.

When you apply ice, do so for approximately 20 minutes at a time, allowing at least an hour between treatments. Repeat this as often as possible for the first 24 to 72 hours. Loading ice into plastic bags is fine, but having soft-pack ice bags in the freezer is markedly more efficient, not to mention a lot less messy. Soft-packs tend to warm up quickly when they contact inflamed skin and joints, but if you have several, you can just keep rotating them. Be careful when applying ice near sensitive nerves (such as those of the spine, or at the back of the knee) or important organs like the eyes and heart.

As well, don't make the mistake of icing something, then following up with a hot bath, which will actually open up the blood vessels and increase swelling.

Compression

Compression—achieved with an elastic bandage—helps reduce swelling, pain and bruising and hasten the healing process, especially when combined with ice and elevation. If you're self-doctoring with an elastic bandage, don't overdo the tension. A compression bandage should be left on for no longer than three hours, unless you are following the advice of a qualified professional. It should never be left on overnight.

Elevation

Elevation serves two purposes. If your foot or another injured body part is elevated, you're not walking around or running on it. (See "Rest," page 137.) More important, however, at least in the short term, when your injured extremity is above your heart there is less pooling of the blood and therefore less swelling. As with ice, when it comes to elevation, sooner is better.

COMMON INJURIES

By following the 13-week RunWalk program, giving sufficient time to warming up and cooling down, watching where you are going and investing in proper footwear, not to mention feeding your body properly and keeping it hydrated, you are going a long way toward preventing injury. Nevertheless, on the theory that it's best to be prepared, the following are parts of the body most commonly affected by running-related injury (The list is from Dr. Tim Noakes and is arranged from the most to the least frequent site of injury.):

> attachment of ligament to bone and tendon to bone
> bones
> muscles
> tendons
> bursae (the fluid-filled sacs between tendons and bones that allow for free movement of tendons over bones)
> blood vessels (both arteries and veins)
> nerves

SUMMARY

If you've been injured, remember the word RICE as a guideline for what you should do.

> **R**est or restrict activity until an accurate diagnosis can be made.
> **I**ce the injury for 20 minutes per hour as often as possible for the first 24–48 hours.
> **C**ompress the injury with an elastic tension bandage (but never too tightly or for too long).
> **E**levate the injured area about the level of the heart.

Within this wide range of possibilities are half a dozen injuries sport medicine practitioners are most commonly called upon to treat, summarized here for your convenience.

Patello-femoral syndrome

Also known as runner's knee (a term coined in the 1970s by running guru and author Dr. George Sheehan), patello-femoral syndrome is characterized by some very specific symptoms, including:

> - localized pain around the kneecap that is not the result of sudden trauma
> - pain in the knee that gets worse over time and often manifests itself after a certain distance
> - pain that comes on if the knee is bent and immobile for a certain period of time, such as when you're sitting in a movie theater

Runner's knee is a huge problem and accounts for about a quarter of all visits to sport medicine clinics. It is a classic overuse injury and occurs at the inner or outer border of the kneecap. Noakes says runner's knee is most commonly caused by excessive ankle pronation (inward rotation of the foot). The foot itself may be at fault, or it may be compensating for an abnormality elsewhere. In any case, the excessive pronation causes a twisting force at the knee, pulling the kneecap out of its correct alignment. Keep pulling on it long enough and you will be looking for ice packs and an aisle seat next time you go to the movies.

Short-term treatment for runner's knee includes the RICE technique, but you can heal it in the long term only if you correct the underlying biomechanical problems causing it. Some doctors may advise surgery; you are well advised to get a second opinion if this treatment is recommended to you.

One way to correct overpronation is to work with your footwear to prevent the foot from twisting. Sometimes a more supportive and/or differently shaped shoe can make a difference; some people need the further help of orthotics (customized foot supports). Orthotics play an important role, and they should be prescribed and built by trained experts. Consult with your doctor or podiatrist about this option.

Iliotibial band syndrome

Runner's knee isn't the only injury that can affect your knees. The iliotibial band is a strip of connective tissue that runs from the hip down the outside of the leg to just below the knee, where it is inserted into the outside of the tibia (shin bone). Repeated bending and straightening of the knee, combined with biomechanical weaknesses, can lead to this connective tissue becoming irritated as it rubs back and forth over the bony outside of the knee, a protuberance known as the femoral condyle. If you've ever had this happen, you can talk with some authority about what it might be like to get shot in the knee: this injury can be extremely painful. In general, the pain may go away with rest but comes on with relentless fury during exercise, when movement causes the iliotibial band to cross the femoral condyle.

Poor shoes, hard running surfaces and training errors have all been cited as possible causes of iliotibial band syndrome, but Macintyre claims it's often a compensatory injury. Noakes agrees, having found that about 70 percent of sufferers have biomechanical structures that inadequately absorb shock. These structures include bowlegs, high arches and rigid feet.

RICE is a good local treatment, but long-term treatment should include softer shoes that can better absorb shock. Avoid hard running surfaces, and cambered roads and hills, both up and down. A good warm-up and stretching program is crucial to prevent (or recover from) iliotibial band syndrome, and gradual adjustments to your training routine may also be required.

If this condition comes on suddenly, ask yourself if you're doing something you didn't do before. Did you change your

....
FACT
....

Running strengthens the joints by improving muscle tone, increasing bone density and increasing the amount of synovial (lubricating) fluid.

running route? Did you just buy new shoes? If so, go back to the old way for a while and see if it makes a difference.

Plantar fasciitis

Plantar fasciitis is less common than iliotibial band syndrome and runner's knee, but it's a pain in the foot for those who get it. Patients commonly complain of what feels like a bruised heel; putting pressure on it hurts.

Actually, the heel itself is not the problem. The plantar fascia is a band of connective tissue running from the heel to the toes; trouble can occur where it attaches to the heel. People who suffer from plantar fasciitis have difficulty when running and when getting out of bed in the morning. You can spot them walking stiffly, because when they put their full weight on their foot the arch stretches out and causes pain.

Plantar fasciitis is thought to be caused by the same thing as runner's knee—excessive pronation. It also tends to occur

VINCE, 50, is a writer who has spent a lifetime indulging in sports, but his endurance needed a boost. Running seemed like the perfect way to increase his cardiovascular conditioning; he reckoned it would make him an even better tennis player and help him keep up with his opponents. Slowly, running took over. "I came to enjoy running. I like the idea that you can do it at your own pace and you don't have to worry about having the right facilities, or opponents or anything."

Then Vince started having shooting pains in his feet. The diagnosis was stress fractures. Instead of running through the pain with painkillers, Vince changed his program and rehabilitated his feet. "I took some time off, went over to cycling for a while and started a stretching program." He avoided running on concrete, opting for soft tracks and park trails instead. As a result, Vince is now back running three times a week for 40 minutes at a stretch.

more commonly in people with high arches. Research so far indicates that overly stiff shoes can exacerbate the condition, as can a sudden increase in the frequency or intensity of training. Plantar fasciitis is a classic overuse injury, and if you get it, it's a sign that your training may be progressing too quickly. Although the 13-week RunWalk program is paced to avoid injury, it may be too much for some people. If you get plantar fasciitis while following the prescribed program, you may be one of them. If that's the case, you will need to back off and take a more gradual approach.

Treatment for plantar fasciitis includes RICE. Consider your footwear carefully; try a softer shoe or perhaps orthotics. Also, try running on softer surfaces. Strengthening and stretching can help. Work on your quadriceps (the big muscles at the front of your upper leg), calf muscles and the small muscles in your feet.

Achilles tendinitis

The Achilles tendon is named for an ancient Greek hero who was considered invulnerable. At birth, his mother dipped him in a special bath that made his skin impregnable. The problem was, she held him by the heel to do it, so that part of his body didn't get the benefit of the magic solution. Achilles went down in the Trojan War when an enemy spear severed the seemingly unimportant tendon running from his calf muscles to his heel. Ever since the poet Homer first immortalized Achilles, the story of his tendon has been used as a metaphor for the weak link in a seemingly impregnable chain. As it turns out, you don't need to sever this tendon to be out of action: a little inflammation—that is, Achilles tendinitis—will do the trick.

Damage to the Achilles tendon can occur quickly, as it did with our Greek hero, or over time, as it usually does with runners. Sufferers first notice a prickly or burning sensation, followed later by a more acute, shooting pain that is especially noticeable when they change direction or run uphill. Over time, the collagen protein fibers of the tendon can break down, and the results can be catastrophic—the tendon may actually snap or rupture. The pain is, as you can imagine, remarkable.

The Achilles tendon is particularly vulnerable as it has a poor blood supply to the area that is more often affected. Add excessive ankle pronation, which tends to cause a whipping action, and the result is tendinitis. Other contributing causes can include constant rubbing of the shoe against the tendon, insufficient warm-up, poor shoe quality or fit, trauma and some kind of heel bone deformity.

Treatment includes RICE and trying a more stable shoe that controls foot motion. Orthotics can help, as can working to increase the flexibility and strength of your feet, calves and shins. Don't be reluctant to take this complaint to a doctor; an untreated Achilles injury can have lasting implications.

Tibial stress syndrome

Sometimes incorrectly referred to as shin splints, tibial stress syndrome is usually caused by minute tears in the muscles where they attach to the shin. The damage can occur in any of three places: anterior (at the front of the tibia—the big bone in your lower leg), posterior (at the back of the tibia) or laterally (along the fibula—the smaller bone in your lower leg). Numerous explanations for these injuries have been put forth, including tightness in the muscles, for which the traditional cure was surgery. Today, researchers blame excessive pronation or too much shock to the bone from repeatedly applied stress. Inadequate flexibility in the ankle—an old injury?—could also be the cause.

Treatment includes RICE, cutting back on running for a time (listen to your body—one to two weeks should do it), orthotics and stretching and strengthening the muscles in the lower leg. Avoid overstriding while running and make sure your shoes provide you with good support and cushioning.

Stress fractures

Stress fractures are very small, incomplete breaks or cracks in bones that result from repeated stress or pounding. Bones repair themselves, of course, but if you knock away at them faster than they can regenerate, they will deteriorate. You can get stress fractures just about anywhere, but runners generally get them in their shins and/or feet. And it's not just small bones that are susceptible; stress fractures in the hip are also possible.

Although repeated pounding is the most common cause of stress fractures, you can also pave the way for them by cheating your body of the nutritional elements it needs to carry on the important job of bone building. (See Chapter 8, Fueling the Body.) Stress fractures do not generally show up on X-rays until healing is well underway. Your doctor *may* order a bone scan to help make the diagnosis, but a physical exam is often sufficient. The key sign of a stress fracture is acute pain that can be pinpointed to a specific area.

Treatment includes RICE and switching away from whatever activity is causing the damage until sufficient healing has taken place to allow a return to that activity. Casting is almost never recommended, though depending on the site and the seriousness of the fracture, immobilization (using crutches) may be an option. Stress fractures can be serious if not treated early and well; deal with them when they first present themselves and you will get back to running sooner. To prevent stress fractures, avoid running on hard surfaces and make sure you have the right shoes for your feet.

Delayed onset muscle soreness (DOMS)

It is not uncommon to feel stiff and sore after you exercise, if you try a new activity or start up again after some time away from it. "Delayed onset muscle soreness, or DOMS," explains Dr. Jim Macintyre, "is caused by microtrauma to tiny blood vessels as a result of an unaccustomed amount of exercise.

The trauma causes the blood vessels to leak and fluid to accumulate." The soreness indicates that you are trying to do too much too soon. Exercise gently until the soreness and swelling decrease, and stretch, cool the affected muscles and elevate your legs.

COMING BACK

Not everyone who takes up running gets a running injury, and if you do, you don't necessarily have to stop training until you are completely healed. Provided your doctor doesn't object, there are a variety of low-impact aerobic activities you can do while injured that will help keep you in the shape to which you have become accustomed. These can include rowing, swimming, pool running, cycling, cross-country skiing or even walking. And if you treat your injuries properly, most will heal in three to four weeks (longer for stress fractures) and you can return to your regular routine.

Don't return to running too soon, however. You want to come back gradually. If you were halfway through the program when you were sidelined and you've now been off for any length of time, consider starting from the beginning. Starting over may not sound like much fun, but remember that elite athletes frequently use a program very much like the 13-week RunWalk program when they are returning from injury layoffs. One general rule is to never increase your activity level by more than 10 percent (time or distance) per week. Follow your doctor's advice and keep the following cautions in mind before resuming your running program:

> Ensure that you have a pain-free range of motion in the injured area.
> Check that the injured side of your body is equal—in terms of strength, endurance, coordination and speed of movement— to your uninjured side, or at least that it performs as well as it did before you were injured.
> Ensure that you are psychologically prepared to return to running and confident you will not be re-injured.

Keep in mind that the injuries discussed in this chapter are only the most common ones runners can acquire. There are others. Pay attention to your aches and pains and seek the advice of a qualified sport medicine practitioner if you have any concerns. Getting in shape is a good thing; hurting or damaging your body in pursuit of this goal is not.

Psychological effects of injuries

Up to this point, we have focused our attention on the physical aspects of rehabilitation from injury. For until recently, much of the focus in sport medicine has been on athletes' *physical* readiness to return to running. However, an injury that prevents you from running can also be a highly emotional experience, one that disrupts your mental health and well-being. And increasingly, medical practitioners are recognizing the importance of helping runners and regular exercisers cope with the psychological effects of their injuries. Without acknowledging and treating the emotional side of an injury, they know they are addressing only part of the problem.

How a person reacts and later deals with an injury varies according to the individual. According to sport psychologist Dr. David Cox, anyone who runs regularly or who has a regular exercise regimen will endure a sometimes lengthy adjustment period after an injury when they are unable to perform at their best. Many psychologists believe there are five stages in this adjustment period: denial and isolation, anger, bargaining, depression and acceptance. As Dr. Cox notes, "This model can be useful in anticipating emotional reactions to injury."

Staying active while injured

For various reasons, some of which have been identified earlier, it is important to stay active while injured. One way is with cross training—a great way to maintain strength and cardio fitness while injured. Cross training also helps fight the injury blues, which are all too common.

TIP

Tips for injured runners
> Seek out positive relationships with empathetic caregivers.
> Educate yourself as to the nature of your injury and the expected course of recovery.
> Develop a rehabilitation program.
> Learn helpful psychological skills, such as goal setting, relaxation, positive self-talk and imagery.
> Prepare yourself for possible setbacks and/or unexpected developments in your recovery.

For anyone who has been forced to take a break from running, or who has lived with someone in this situation, being sidelined with an injury can be fraught with frustration. But it doesn't have to be this way. Recovering from an injury can be seen as an opportunity to try a new activity and to strengthen areas of the body you may have otherwise neglected. If you cross train while injured, it's also likely you will be more patient and able to take a more gradual approach to returning to running. Starting back too soon or too quickly because you're anxious about losing fitness or gaining weight regularly results in re-injury.

Pool running

Besides swimming, cycling and walking, why not try pool running? It may not seem like the most exciting activity, but running in a pool is a great way to stay fit while nursing an injury. It's also a safe and effective way to add an extra run to your schedule and to avoid overuse injuries common to increases in running time and intensity.

Tips for running in water

The idea with pool running is to develop a proper running technique—using quick turnover of your arms and legs to allow you to stay afloat and move from one end of the pool to the other. It is not a race to get to the other end, but it is not a walk in the water, either. As you develop your technique:

> Try to mirror your running gait.
> Avoid a bicycle movement with your legs—extend your quadriceps forward rather than upward, and focus on pulling strongly back through the water with the hamstrings.
> Maintain an upright position and avoid leaning forward too much.
> Keep your head comfortably above water.
> Avoid dog-paddling; keep your shoulders relaxed and move your arms straight forward and backward in the water.

> Break the surface of the water in front with the fingertips and in back with the elbows . . . a strong arm action is very helpful.
> Concentrate on keeping your elbows close to your body (to avoid a sideways motion).

RETURNING TO RUNNING AFTER A SIGNIFICANT MEDICAL PROBLEM

If you want to return to running after suffering a significant medical problem such as a heart attack, hip replacement surgery or cancer, it's essential to do so under the direction of your health care provider. Even if you were a regular exerciser prior to your health problems, it is important to heed the advice of your doctor.

The following are some commonly asked running-related questions from people wanting to know if—and how—they

LYNN is a former Canadian Olympian and bronze-medal winner in the 3,000 meters at 1984's Los Angeles Olympics. Over the years, Lynn has overcome iliotibial band syndrome and numerous stress fractures. Leading up to the L.A. Olympics, Lynn was again devastated by a stress fracture that left her unable to run.

"During previous periods of injury, I cross trained using swimming and cycling to maintain fitness. While these activities left me aerobically fit, I was exercising different muscles from those used in running. So when it was suggested that I try running in water, I was open to it."

With Lynn's sights set on the Olympic Games, she was determined to make her new training regimen work. After a few weeks, she developed a comfortable and effective technique. Lynn trained exclusively in the water for eight weeks before she ran again on land. Four weeks after coming out of the pool, she ran a personal best in the 3,000 meters and set a new Canadian record. Lynn attributed her recovery to running in water.

Lynn

can return to running, with responses from sport medicine specialist Dr. Jack Taunton.

Q *Can I return to running after my injury?*
A For someone who is recovering from a significant medical problem, such as hip replacement surgery, or who is constantly plagued with sore knees, running may not be the best activity to take up again after an injury. Rather, walking, swimming or cycling may be better options.

Q *I consistently have sore knees, even though I wear proper shoes and have been correctly fitted for orthotics. Can I begin a running program again or should I try another sport?*
A Before giving up on running, try building up your quadriceps strength with drop squats, then build up gradually through the SportMedBC RunWalk program.

Q *I recently underwent hip replacement surgery. Will I ever be able to return to a regular running routine?*
A No, not if you want your hip to last a long time. It's important that you try another sport, such as cycling or swimming.

Q *I suffer from arthritis, is it okay for me to run?*
A It depends on the site of the arthritis. Improve your strength if it involves the hip, knees and/or ankles, then cycle, swim and, as the inflammation is controlled, try the SportMedBC RunWalk program.

CHAPTER 9 SUMMARY

1. Stick with your training schedule: don't try to skip ahead, especially in the first few weeks of the program.
2. Listen to your body: if you feel pain, back off your training and seek advice from a medical practitioner.

3. Promptly attend to injuries: use the RICE treatment and seek advice from a medical practitioner if the injury seems serious or if pain persists.
4. Modify your training when injured or ill. Don't try to "run through" an injury or illness, but stay active while injured by cross training, swimming, pool running or cycling, which will take stress off your legs and help maintain your fitness.
5. Avoid poor shoes, hard or uneven running surfaces and training errors, which are most frequently cited as contributing factors to the more common running injuries.

10

Preparing for
a 10-k Event

....

YOU HAVE taken your fitness level to new heights, have become a
consistent and dedicated runner and now it's time to start planning
to run your first 10-k race. Running a race is an exciting and exhil-
arating experience. Tens of thousands of people like you training
on roads, trails and tracks are striving toward completing the 10-k
distance.

The most important "to-do" item is to line up your training so
the end of the 13-week RunWalk program coincides with race day.
Place your race day as the last training session of week 13. Then
work backward to determine when your training needs to start.

Bruce Angus, 35, a self-professed "amateur professional" runner, has been entering events on and off for the better part of
20 years. After years of trial and error, of good finishes and bad,
he's learned a lot about event preparation. "The first thing you want
to do is make sure you've done all your training before race day," he
says with a chuckle. (Don't laugh. You'd be surprised how many
people think they can train half-heartedly—or even enthusiasti-
cally—for a week or two before a race and then go the distance.)

Before competing, Angus is like a race-car driver: he likes to scope out the track and get a feel for the environment he's going to be running in. "I like to drive, cycle or even run the track before the race. If you've been through the course, you have a clear understanding of the terrain and you can visualize moving through it, where you're going to pass people. It's also good to know what kind of surface it is, whether it's grass or gravel or pavement. The kind of surface and the distance will dictate the kind of footwear you're going to choose."

Whatever your motivation for entering an event, a few moments of planning can make all the difference in your enjoyment of it.

BEFORE THE EVENT

Identify the 10-k event you want to train for and commit to the date before you start your 13-week RunWalk training program. You can often find race applications at local running stores, at community centers and fitness clubs as well as online. An added benefit of signing up early is that entry fees often increase significantly as race day draws near, and some of the larger events do not take entries on that day.

In the week before the event, your focus will be on getting mentally and practically prepared for race day. Your last week of training tapers toward race day and provides for some rest in the last few days before the run. Squeezing in more training at that stage won't get you any fitter. Try to get some good sleep in this final week. Chances are that you will be nervous the night before the race, which often leads to a restless night. This can easily be overcome if you manage to get several good sleeps earlier in the week.

Throughout your training, but especially in the last week, eat well. Everyday eating is ultimately more important than the pre-event meal, so making proper food choices in the weeks prior to event day will help you. The pre-race meal cannot compensate for a poor training diet, and the energy from

Don't worry if you don't
sleep well the night
before a race. It's more
important to get a good
night's sleep two nights
before the race.

that meal will not reach the muscles in time to help your performance (except in endurance races of three hours or more). What will make a big difference is staying hydrated, so steer clear of alcohol in the day or two prior to the event. If you do have a drink, make sure you also consume plenty of water. It's important that your body is well hydrated before the race.

Exploring the racecourse can help you prepare mentally. Check out the map of the course or, better yet, take some time to walk, drive or cycle it prior to event day. Don't be tempted to run or walk the entire course before the event: save your best effort for the big day.

Finally, pick up your race package in the days leading up to the event. The race package will consist of your race number, a timing chip if the event uses this type of automated system and perhaps some goodies from various race sponsors. Picking up your race package and soaking in the event's atmosphere can be a great way to get excited for the race.

Pre-event checklist

> Rest up, especially in the last 72 hours before the race.
> Plan healthy meals on a regular schedule and stay hydrated.
> Pick up your race package.
> Review a map of the course (or drive the actual course the day before) to know where the bathrooms, medical tent and water stations are.

DAY-BEFORE PREPARATIONS

Try to make the day before your event as restful as possible so you're not using a lot of energy. But a little planning ahead can reduce your anxiety on race day.

Check the weather forecast and plan what you're going to wear: be careful not to overdress. Lay out your clothing and your running shoes. To keep warm at the start, plan to wear an old sweatshirt or garbage bag that you can discard once you get underway. Make sure your running shoes are well worn in. The biggest mistake you can make is using a new pair of running shoes on race day.

In addition to laying out the clothes and shoes you plan to wear, it is also a good idea to pack a bag that includes a few essential race-day items (for example, a change of clothes, socks and a pair of comfortable shoes, a towel, water bottle, sunblock and light snack) and whatever else you think you might need straight after the race. Investigate whether a gear check will be available; if it is, assemble these items in a bag you can easily identify. You might also want to pack some toilet paper, as pre-race toilet visits on-site are often met with empty paper dispensers.

Pin your race number on your running shirt. If you have any medical issues such as asthma, allergies, diabetes, hypertension or other cardiovascular or health problems, it is a good idea to jot a brief medical history and list any medications you take regularly on the back of your number. This is the first place medical personnel will check in the event of an emergency. If your event is using a timing chip, attach the chip as directed to your shoe with the zip-tie provided. Be sure it is secure and doesn't flap around.

Once you've organized your clothing, plan where to meet up with your family and friends. With many thousands of runners taking part in large events, the finish area can get very busy. Decide on a meeting place that everyone can find when you have finished the race.

Finally, decide what you are going to eat before the race. Most runners tend to stick to foods they're familiar with and enjoy eating. Pasta is a great meal the night before the event, as it is full of carbohydrates and is easily digested. You will also need to think about what you will eat first thing on race day. Timing is important. If you are able to eat two or more hours before running, plan to eat a small high-carbohydrate meal that is low in fat and has a small amount of protein for lasting energy. Some possible choices include:

> low-fat yogurt with low-fat granola and raisins
> a whole-grain bagel with peanut butter and honey
> healthy, ready-to-eat cold cereal with low-fat milk or soy milk
> oatmeal with 1 percent milk and a piece of fruit

If you only have an hour or so before the run, plan to drink a liquid meal such as a yogurt-and-fruit smoothie or a meal-replacement drink. Sport energy bars are alternatives, but be sure to choose a bar that provides at least 1 ounce (30 grams) of carbohydrates and no more than 0.28 ounces (8 grams) of protein.

Day-before checklist

> Prepare a bag with your race clothing and a change of clothes the night before the event.
> Write a list of any medications or allergies on the back of your race number, then pin the number to your shirt. If your event uses them, attach your timing chip to your shoe.
> Eat a carbohydrate-rich meal, such as pasta, the night before the race and another small high-carb meal just before the event.
> Drink lots and drink often the day before the race. You want to be well hydrated.
> Double-check the start time and location of the race and take one last look at the map of the course.

> Decide on a meeting point with your friends and family after the race.

Pack your bag the night before with the following items:
> running shoes (and extra shoelaces) with timing chip, if provided
> running clothing, including your race number attached with safety pins
> towel and toilet paper
> sunblock
> water bottle
> race information
> cash

RACE DAY

On the big day, you're likely to be excited and nervous. Note the time the event starts and plan to arrive on-site at least an hour before. Allow plenty of time to park, visit the restroom (they will be very crowded) and get to the start line.

Take time to warm up properly at the start (approximately 20 minutes prior to the start of the event). Even if you want to conserve energy for the race, skipping your warm-up is a bad idea. To keep your heart rate up, move around or jog in place until "the gun goes off." As you're waiting, be sure to drink 1 to 2 cups water, 10 to 15 minutes prior to the start. Also, go easy on the coffee. You will want to avoid foods and drinks that might upset your stomach.

In most races, participants line up according to how fast they plan to complete the event so stay out of the front row, as it is usually reserved for the most elite runners. Remember that your goal is to finish the race, and you don't want to get swept away at the start at a pace that is way too fast for you. Some events have pacers based on your projected finishing time; look to see if there are people holding any of these signs and, if you have a goal time, position yourself around them.

TIP

Set your alarm clock and double-check it. If you're staying in a hotel, request a wake-up call, just to be safe.

Water loss (sweat) over a 10-k distance is very individual. However, environmental factors such as heat and rain will play a big role in sweat rates.

If weather is an issue, try to keep warm and dry as best you can. If you are concerned about getting a chill while waiting for the start, wear the T-shirt or sweatshirt you've brought to discard, until just before the run begins. Many race organizers will collect the discarded clothes and donate them to a local charity. Another idea is to tear holes for your head and arms in an old garbage bag and pull it over your body.

After the gun goes off

Be patient at the start, as it may take a little while to cross the start line. If you are concerned about an accurate time, use your own sport watch. If the event uses timing chips, yours will activate as you cross the start line and keep timing until you cross the finish line. This "chip time" is an accurate measure of the time it took you to complete the course.

Start at a pace that you can maintain throughout the entire 10 k. It should feel relatively easy for the first couple of kilometers. If you go out too fast, you will be miserable for most of the race and risk not finishing at all, so make sure you don't run faster than usual because you are trying to keep up

Ranji

AS a race-event organizer, Ranji loves arriving at the course before anyone else is there. "There is a calmness on the road that I really enjoy," she exclaims. "Once people start to arrive, the atmosphere starts to change." Her major advice to participants is to "know the course. The day before the event, follow the course on a map—drive it; don't run it. Also, get to know where the bathrooms and water stations are located so you don't start to panic mid-race."

Ranji has organized races all over British Columbia, in all kinds of weather. She advises participants to dress in layers because the weather can change so drastically. "Sometimes the morning starts off pretty wet, but 30 minutes into the race the sun is shining and it's pretty warm outside. Dressing in layers is a great way to not overheat while running."

with someone else. Once you settle into your pace, enjoy the ambiance and the scenery, be courteous and avoid sudden stops and changes in direction and run in a safe and predictable manner. There will be a lot of others in the race, making it easy to trip or stumble into another runner's path. If you are trying to pass someone, make sure you are a couple of strides ahead before cutting across. If you are going slower than the rest of the pack, try to steer a course to the right and allow faster runners a clear path around you. Finally, follow the course. Cutting corners to shorten the distance you have to cover is cheating. Pride yourself on completing the entire course.

At the aid stations on the course, don't forget to drink. One third to a half a cup of water is recommended every 15 to 20 minutes during the run. Try not to drop your water cup on the course where someone might trip on it. Use the bins provided or, at the very least, toss your cup well to the side.

After the event

You may be exhausted and want to stop or overjoyed and want to savor the moment when you reach the finish line, but keep moving. There are lots of runners converging on this point, and it can become a real bottleneck. Don't jump the queue, especially if timing chips are not being used, because the order you arrive at the finish line will affect the overall results. Listen for directions from race officials and go with the flow.

Once you are through the finish line, take time to cool down properly. Keep your muscles active for 10 to 15 minutes after you finish, and while you are still warm get into your stretching routine. This should involve some gentle exercises— for your calves, quadriceps, hamstrings and gluteals.

While you're stretching, help yourself to the water and refreshments available at the finish area. Bagels, bananas and energy bars are all good choices. Replenish the fluids and nutrients you expended during the event and be sure to put your litter and banana peels in the bins provided.

TIP

If you have some energy to spare in the last part of the race, pick out runners ahead of you to catch and pass. This is an enjoyable mind game that will help keep you motivated until the finish line.

Most of all, celebrate your accomplishments. Once the event is over, take time to congratulate yourself and celebrate with friends and family. Wear your event T-shirt with pride; you'll be surprised how many conversations with complete strangers it will spark. Once the dust settles, pick another 10-k event and start the process all over again. Enjoy the road ahead!

Day-of checklist

> Two to three hours before the race begins, start hydrating and eat a small high-carbohydrate meal that is low in fat and has a small amount of protein.
> Begin to warm up 20 minutes before the start of the event.
> Prepare for any type of weather by wearing a garbage bag or old clothes to keep warm.
> Pace yourself.
> Relax and have fun!

CHAPTER 10 SUMMARY

1. Choose your 10-k event before you begin the 13-week Run-Walk program so you can focus on your goal each week and complete your training before the race.
2. Getting enough rest, eating properly, staying hydrated and studying the course in the weeks before the event will go a long way toward making your race day a success.
3. Planning and organizing ahead of time what you will wear, how you will get to the event and what you will do afterward will free you up to relax and enjoy the race.
4. Pace yourself throughout the race and be sure to stop for water at each of the aid stations.
5. Celebrate your accomplishment, then start thinking about your next running goal.

11

What's Next?

························

WHEN YOU have completed the 13-week RunWalk program, you will likely think of yourself as a different person. You will have taken yourself to a new level of fitness, and probably given your self-confidence a boost as well. You will know that if you set your mind to something, you can achieve it. If you have trained with others, you will doubtless have made new friends outside your traditional circle. But when the program is over, you may find yourself asking, "Now what?"

From a physiological standpoint, your successful completion of the program brings you both good news and bad. The good news is that the cardiovascular (heart and lung) fitness you have worked so patiently to develop over the past 13 weeks is relatively easy to maintain. All you have to do is carry on doing what you have been doing—exercising aerobically three times a week for 30 to 40 minutes. You do not have to perpetually push yourself further. If, however, you want to continue to improve your fitness level, you're going to have to continue challenging your body. One way to do this is to follow the 13-week Run Faster program found in Appendix C of this book (page 198). You will notice that it offers additional challenges, including hill-repeat sessions and interval training. But remember: do not begin the intermediate program until you have completed the 13-week RunWalk program and, even then, only if you are running regularly. Otherwise you will risk getting injured.

The bad news is that if you've thought of completing the program as the end of the road, the fitness you have worked so hard to attain will slowly seep away, like water into sand. By the end of a month, it will be vastly diminished. You may find it unfair that you worked so hard and then don't get to rest on your laurels for a while, but that's the way it is. Your body will return to the state it was in before you started the program.

Some people don't mind. They may have taken on the program simply to see if they could do it or because friends challenged them. Sometimes these people drift away from fitness altogether and never come back. It's a personal choice—though not a very healthy one.

Other people find that when they get to the end of the program and don't have a schedule to follow, their motivation slips out the door. It's not so much a choice: they're just lost without a script, and before they realize it, they're out of shape again.

If this happens to you, or if a life event—a sickness in the family, say, or a crisis at work—prevents you from maintaining your current level of fitness, you can always start over again. It isn't as bad as it sounds. You already know that in your hands you have both the prescription and the cure. You can simply go back to the beginning, start over and in 13 weeks you'll be back on top. Nor will you be alone. Many people who let their fitness slide after completing the program eventually become unhappy about huffing and puffing like an old steam locomotive every time they have to sprint for the bus and return to the program many months later. It is infinitely better to start again than to quit for good.

However, by following the program, most of you will have found that you actually enjoy your new level of fitness and would like to do whatever is necessary to maintain it. To begin, taking a few days off after you complete the program isn't going to hurt your fitness level at all. Quite the opposite, in fact; your body will probably be grateful for the opportunity to recover, especially if you were training for a running event and your program culminated in a 10-k run. As the week following the race or program completion goes by, however, you should start thinking about how you are going to follow up and get into a regular program of maintenance.

There are a number of ways to stay in top form. You can simply continue with your current time commitment of three 30- to 40-minute sessions a week, which should be relatively easy because your body is already programmed to do it. If you find the longer sessions too onerous or time consuming, you can stick to half-hour sessions during the week, provided you make time for at least one session of 45 to 60 minutes on the weekend. You can adjust the time you spend training to suit your schedule; just keep in mind that the key to maintaining fitness is frequency and intensity—and that it is a lot less work to maintain a fitness level than to establish one; working out for even 20 minutes is better than nothing. Or you can train by engaging in 10- to 15-minute "spurts" of exercise throughout the day. If you don't feel like running at all, a fast walk will suffice to get your heart rate up and help you maintain a healthy level of fitness.

If you find your motivation slipping away, sign up for one of the many running and walking events in your community. There are runners everywhere these days, and most of them love getting together. The events they attend are partly a way to gauge progress and partly a way to socialize. Your local running shoe store or community center will likely have a schedule of such events. As well, walking clubs abound, and their weekly activities are often listed in local newspapers.

If you complete the program and decide that running isn't for you, don't despair. Running isn't for everyone, which is probably a good thing, because if it were, some running paths

FACT

A 1997 study by researchers at Stanford University showed that people who exercise, maintain a healthy weight and don't smoke are half as likely to become disabled by age 75 as people who don't have these habits.

would get very crowded. Still, not loving to run shouldn't mean retreating to the sofa and the remote control. As discussed in Chapter 7, there are all kinds of other enjoyable aerobic activities. Cycling, swimming, cross-country skiing and hiking are excellent alternatives to running, as are in-line skating, kayaking, group fitness classes, walking or even just putting in some time on the stair climber at your local gym.

The important thing is that you find an aerobic activity you enjoy. The more you enjoy it, the more likely you are to find the time for it. Furthermore, although you need to keep some kind of aerobic activity at the center of your fitness plan, you might like to sample some anaerobic, stop-and-go sports as well. If you enjoy games, you might try soccer, squash, softball, volleyball, tennis, basketball, hockey or badminton. Some of these activities may look as though they involve a lot of standing around, but keep in mind that you'll get as much out of them as you're prepared to invest. Badminton can be a leisurely activity, or you can work hard and break a real

AFTER three years of running, Lisa was in the best shape of her life, but she heard the siren of other activities calling her name. "My boyfriend's a climber, and he took me out to this mountain," she says. "There was no pressure or anything, but I wanted to keep up with him and his friends. When I reached the last 10 feet (3 meters) I froze. My boyfriend helped me down to a ledge, and I waited for the panic to subside. He told me it didn't matter that I'd only managed to get near the top, but I knew I'd have to try again.

"It was easier the next time partly because I knew what to expect. I crawled up and put my hand on the highest point and then scrambled back down. I think it was the hardest thing I've ever done." She still likes running but has caught the climbing bug as she exclaims, "There are a lot of mountains to climb out there."

sweat—it's up to you. The important thing is to get and stay fit by doing activities you enjoy.

When approaching any sport, remember the three rules of exercise—moderation, consistency and rest—and don't expect to be an expert right away. Each sport requires unique skills and it will take you a while to acquire them. Each time you take up a new activity, you'll find there are as many comfort-zone barriers to cross as you are willing to take on. As well, you will invariably reach plateaus of competence that only patience and practice will take you beyond. If you're having trouble progressing, take lessons. Or, seek assistance from a more experienced participant: every sport has a dedicated core of enthusiasts who are glad to help out newcomers and show them the ropes.

In addition to taking part in aerobic and anaerobic activities, it's a good idea to do some strength training. This can involve weights or circuit training. If you want to increase your strength and also push some comfort-zone barriers, try climbing.

No matter which activities you choose, it's essential to prepare yourself properly. This includes warming up and cooling down, eating nutritious food, wearing suitable clothing and equipment and staying aware of the potential for injuries. In other words, the basics you learned in this book are relevant to all the activities you may take up.

DECIDING ON YOUR NEXT CHALLENGE

Regardless of whether you want to maintain your current fitness level, diversify your exercise program or improve your 10-k time, the important point to remember is that you are already a fitness success. By now, you understand that setting a goal and having a clear plan of how to get there are the keys to success.

Many of you may already have your next fitness goal in mind, but for those who don't, you may want to consider some

FACT

Over the past 17 years, more than 75,000 Run-Walk participants have successfully completed a 10-k running event.

of the following questions to assist you in establishing your next athletic milestone:

> How long have you been maintaining a regular running routine?
> How much time do you have to commit to your exercise program?
> Have you been injury free for the duration of your 13-week RunWalk program?
> Have you enjoyed your running program enough to continue or increase the distance or intensity?
> Do you feel mentally and physically ready for another fitness challenge?
> Are you bored with running? Do you feel the need to try another athletic activity?

TRAINING TO RUN FASTER

If you have maintained a regular running schedule for at least a year, have been free of injury for several weeks and want to increase the intensity of your training, you may be ready to embark on the new challenge of running faster. The goal of an improved 10-k race time is exciting and quite different from the sole objective of completing a 10-k event. Essential to achieving the goal of an improved race time is a diverse and well-organized training program.

Employing a variety of training techniques will both improve your fitness and help you maintain motivation. Interval training, tempo running, hill and fartlek training are the four general running workouts used by successful runners to build strength and improve speed. Most running experts suggest a weekly schedule that includes one or more speed and strength workouts. If you're a beginning runner, try incorporating one speed workout a week into your running program for the first six to eight weeks. If you already run three times a week, make one of those runs a speed-training session.

Once you have completed approximately eight consecutive

speed-training workouts over the course of eight weeks, and if you are not injured, you may want to introduce a second speed session into your weekly running schedule. The second session, or speed workout, should be different from the first session. For example, if your first eight weeks of speed training included one hill-training session a week, the next session you incorporate might be a fartlek or interval workout.

Like your 13-week RunWalk program, consistency is necessary to improve speed. Given that determination can wane for even the most focused individuals, finding a training partner with similar goals is a good way to improve your motivation and the likelihood of staying on track. If fitness levels vary, speed training can be easily modified to accommodate even the most diverse training groups. By doing shorter speed intervals and regrouping during your rest breaks, groups are able to provide each other with the support and motivation needed to complete demanding workouts.

Hill training

Running up hills builds muscle and cardiovascular endurance and makes a good transition to speed work. Hills also add challenge to more advanced workouts. And hill training is easy to adapt to groups of runners with varying speeds and endurance levels. Remember, you need to treat each hill-training segment as an individual workout and recover before repeating it.

When running up a hill, try not to lean forward; focus on keeping your balance, shortening your leg stride, lifting your knees a little higher and keeping those arms pumping. Before you know it, you will be going down the other side. Use gravity as much as possible and lengthen your stride to keep your hips over your feet.

In planning your hill-training session, choose a hill that is at least 110 yards (100 meters) long and not too steep. You want a hill with a gentle incline that you can run up, not one

FACT

Among cancer survivors who responded to a 1997 University of Utah nursing survey, 90 percent said exercise made them feel more relaxed and refreshed, and 94 percent said it made them feel better about their overall health.

that's too steep. Your hill repeats can be based on time or distance; it's up to you. For example: run hard up the hill for 45 seconds, stop and regroup with your training partners, then jog back down to the start of the hill at an easy pace that allows you to catch your breath. Repeat five to seven times, depending on your fitness level. A word of caution: if you haven't caught your breath by the time you reach the bottom of the hill, you are pushing yourself too hard. It's a good idea to use this as a gauge for how hard you are working. You want to push yourself, but you also want to live to run another day. After about eight weeks, gradually increase your number of hill segments.

Regardless of the type of speed session, always make sure you start your run with at least a 10-minute warm-up at an easy pace. After completing the speed session, it's also a good idea to do a 10-minute cool-down at an easy pace. By including an easy pace before and after a speed session, you are able to warm up and loosen your muscles.

If there aren't any hills in your neighborhood, there are alternatives to building strength and endurance. A few suggestions:

> Treadmill workouts, where you elevate the machine to a 7 percent grade, are a great way to simulate hill running. Depending on the machine, you can do pre-programmed workouts or manually adjust the speed so that your workouts mirror those done on land, as outlined above.

> Bike or step machine intervals are great workouts. Warm up for 10 minutes, increase the intensity for four or five minutes, then recover. After a few sessions, try adding a second repeat to the workout.

> Bleacher steps at your neighborhood baseball field are a challenging and fun way to build leg strength. Warm up, run up the steps at a difficult pace, then walk back down—consider this one set. Gradually increase the number of sets as your strength improves. Remember, if you are still out of breath at the bottom of the stairs, you're pushing yourself too hard.

Interval training

This type of training is a combination of running at a faster than normal pace and walking during the recovery stage. The goal is to increase your capacity to carry oxygen through your system and improve your muscle endurance. You will be running at a slightly higher speed for a short period, followed by a recovery period in which you will walk or jog slowly. You can measure your intervals by time or distance; it's up to you.

Remember to begin each speed-training session with a 10-minute warm-up and end each session with a 10-minute cool-down, followed by some easy stretches. Warm-up and cool-down running is done at an easy speed that allows your muscles to prepare for and recover from the intensity of speed training.

If speed training is new for you, you may want to start with two minutes at your goal race pace, followed by two minutes easy. The two minutes easy is your recovery period where you can walk or jog easy. The two minutes of hard running followed by two minutes of easy running or walking makes up one set. Try three sets for the first three weeks before gradually introducing a fourth and fifth set. For beginners or those new to speed work, don't attempt any more than five sets for the first six to eight months of speed training.

Deciding the distance or time of each workout is up to you. Some runners may want to stick with the same workout for a few months, but for others this approach may become boring. Usually it's a good idea to vary your workouts to keep things interesting and help maintain motivation. Other interval workouts for beginners include

> five minutes hard with 2½ minutes easy. Repeat three times, gradually building to five sets

OR

> three 1-k repeats with a rest period that is approximately half of the acceleration time

Remember, the goal of your rest period is to recover from the hard session so that your breathing can return almost to normal. If you are unable to catch your breath between intervals you are pushing yourself too hard. If this is the case, ease off a little during the intense periods. It takes time to understand how hard to push yourself. Also, how you feel can vary from one run to the next. Outside factors such as wind, rain, heat—as well as stress and sleep—play a role in how hard and fast you can run on a given day. It's always better to start easy so that you can push yourself at the end. By going out too hard, you could end the interval or session feeling like you cannot run another step.

Fartlek training

Fartleks are a series of random bursts done during a continuous walk or run. These bursts can range anywhere from 20 seconds to three minutes and are performed every two to four minutes. Their duration and speed is up to you. But the emphasis should be on running for significant periods at a pace faster than your normal training and racing paces. Each

IT took a move all the way across North America to get Lynn into running, but now that she's started, she says she's never going to stop. "After I moved, I wanted to meet people who shared the same kind of interests I did," says the 29-year-old dietitian. A competitive swimmer in her youth, Lynn not only wanted new friends, she wanted the friends to be fit and active people like her. She heard about a running clinic and signed up.

"It's been a great experience, and I've met such a variety of people. They're my friends now, so I don't know what I'd do if I didn't go running. We have a running club, and we meet every Saturday. Lynn supplements her running with other activities, such as swimming and in-line skating. "I'm aiming for a balance because it seems to be more in keeping with my lifestyle. There are also health reasons for doing other sports. As well, if I run all the time and don't do anything else, I get bored."

hard effort is followed by a recovery stage, when the pace is reduced to a point where breathing and pulse rate return to near-normal resting rate. Still, the key is to keep moving. This type of workout is well suited for trail running over varied terrain.

Before starting your fartlek session, remember to warm up for 10 minutes and to include a 10-minute cool-down upon completing the speed session. Beginners can start with one minute hard followed by one minute easy. Try this 10 times to start with. After six weeks, gradually build up to 12 and then 15 repeats. Another suggestion is to use landmarks such as telephone poles as indicators for speeding up and slowing down. For example: run hard for two telephone poles, then easy for two poles. Repeat seven times and gradually increase to 15 repeats.

Tempo training

Tempo running is when you maintain a continuous pace that is faster than your easy run, but one you can maintain for up to an hour if it were a race. Tempo runs teach the body to run faster before fatiguing, and, like the other speed sessions described in this section, can be done based on time or distance. Beginners might want to start a tempo run that is about 2 miles long (just over 3 kilometers), or 15 to 18 minutes in length. After six weeks of successful training, add ³⁄₄ mile (about 1 kilometer), or seven minutes every couple of weeks until you reach 3³⁄₄ miles (6 kilometers), or 25 minutes. Remember to include your 10-minute warm-up and cool-down before and after every tempo training session. Stretching should also be done for about 10 to 15 minutes at the end of each run.

TRAINING TO RUN FARTHER

If you have completed the 13-week RunWalk program, continue to enjoy running and want to increase the duration of your runs, you may be interested in training for a half or full marathon. These distances are within many people's reach, as long as they train correctly, using all the same basic principles we have advocated in the *Beginning Runner's Handbook*.

But before you jump into a more intense training program, there are a few things you need to think about. If your goal is to run a full marathon, it's important to know that most seasoned runners suggest completing a half-marathon training program before attempting the 26.2-mile (42-kilometer) full-marathon distance. In order to be ready to begin the SportMed 26-week training program, Canadian Olympian Lynn Kanuka suggests that you have run consistently three times a week for at least the past six months.

SportMedBC's *Marathon and Half-Marathon: The Beginner's Guide* will pilot a sedentary person from inactivity through to finishing a half or full marathon in 26 weeks, less time if you have just successfully completed the 13-week RunWalk training. You will have three training sessions each week for the first few months, each of which will take about an hour to complete. As with all SportMed publications, this book will help you get across the finish line, well prepared and injury free.

THE RACE IS ON

Numerous people who complete the 13-week RunWalk program probably knew even before they started that running was the sport for them. Some will use running as a release and always do it alone. Others will think of it as an important adjunct to their social life—a way to make new friends no matter where they go. Many of these people will join running groups and in a few years will be talking about the "thousands" of miles they have run and the dozens of events they have entered. Still others will want above all to race.

There are a number of good reasons for entering races, but the main one should always be because they are fun. There's a great sense of camaraderie around these events, and some runners go just because they love to meet up with the kinds of people who participate in them. Some high-profile races include the *Vancouver Sun* Run™ in British Columbia; the Great North Run in Newcastle, England; Round the Bays in Auckland, New Zealand; the City2Surf in Sydney, Australia; the Bloomsday 12-k in Spokane, Washington; the Peachtree Road Race in Atlanta, Georgia, and the Bay to Breakers in San Francisco—but there are a host of others. These events attract beginning runners and people who have been racing for years. Few of the participants will care much what your time is; they are interested only in their own—and in having fun.

Such events can also be educational. Races are often preceded by running clinics at which expert runners, doctors and physiologists host forums on various running-related topics. What's more, running equipment manufacturers often set up booths to promote their products, so the events also serve as miniature trade fairs and conferences.

Although only one person can cross the finish line first, there's a general consensus that anyone who competes in a race wins simply by taking part. What's more, many races now have separate categories that allow entrants to test their mettle against people their own age. For example, you could come in 62nd or 178th overall, but still wind up fifth in the 45- to 50-year-old group. Still, you don't have to get caught up in competing—just enjoy yourself.

You might also want to experiment with different distances. There are lots of 5-k and 10-k "fun runs." If you find you enjoy participating in them, you can build up to the half-marathon training program outlined in *Marathon and Half-Marathon: The Beginner's Guide* and perhaps enter longer-distance events. But try to be sure long-distance running is what you really want before subjecting yourself to the rigors associated with it. Marathon running is not for everybody any more than every climber needs to scale Mount Everest. If you get into a race that's over your head and halfway through have to pull over with nausea and cramps, you're not likely to want to come back. You'll also be exposing

FACT

There are 1,007 listed
10-k races that take place
worldwide. Every year
there are over 250 char-
ity races across North
America.

yourself to the possibility of injury. The best strategy is to pick a race that's well within your comfort zone and give yourself a chance to complete it.

Providing motivation is one of the biggest reasons to enter a race—maybe the best one. Having a race date set on your calendar can get you to lace up your runners and go, even when your heart says to unlace and sit. Having told all your friends you're going to do it, you won't want everyone asking you how you did and then have to explain that you "didn't feel like it." In racing, success also breeds success. If you do well, you'll be further motivated to train harder and do even better the next time.

If you've been cross training, you may want to think about competing in duathlons or triathlons. As their names imply, these events include more than one sport. Duathlons usually consist of running and cycling. In triathlons, you get to start with a bracing swim, then cycle, then run. The lengths of these events, like those of running events, vary considerably. A short-course duathlon can feature a 5-k run followed by a 20-k bike ride, capped off with another 5-k run, whereas an Iron-man triathlon can include a 2.4-mile (4-k) swim, a 112-mile (180-k) bike ride and then a full marathon (26.2 miles/42 k). They don't call it Ironman for nothing!

Charity runs

Charity running programs are a great way to stay motivated. You can participate in walks and runs and raise money for a wide variety of charities doing work in such areas as health, including cancer; poverty; and abuse. For example, the Run for the Cure is a national 10-k race that has raised millions of dollars to support breast cancer research. These races help to increase enthusiasm by providing runners with two targets to aim for: a reachable training goal and a measurable fundrais-ing goal in support of a cause they believe in. And there are two ways to run for charity, either securing your own place in an event and choosing to raise money for a charity by making a donation, or approaching a charity and running for their official team at a major event.

Charitable organizations will pre-purchase spots to guarantee runners a place in the race. In exchange for agreeing to raise a minimum amount of money—up to $2,500—runners receive an entry to the event and often training advice leading up to the race, exclusive team clothing and support around the course by the charity's cheerers. It's amazing what a difference having your own cheering squad can make! Even if your body is tired, the support and encouragement keeps you motivated until the end. The organizations also help with your fundraising by giving every runner the opportunity to create their own online Web page where friends and family can donate. You can fill your homepage with photos, training logs,

Andy

ANDY is six-foot-two and 220 pounds (1.8 meters and 99 kilograms). Before embarking on his first half marathon, this 40-year-old was concerned that his large frame would be a barrier to achieving his running goal. Andy had always thought of marathoners as people with extremely slight frames. However, using the 13-week RunWalk program and with the help of the guys at the local running store, Andy reworked the 13-week schedule for a 10-k race to incorporate a longer run each weekend in order to prepare him for the 13.1-mile (21-kilometer) half-marathon distance. An additional inspiration for Andy was his friend Seth, who had recently had a near-death experience, underwent a liver transplant and had just completed a full marathon.

Andy's commitment and perseverance in completing the half-marathon training program paid off. He had no problem finishing his race, and he did it in a much faster time than he had thought possible. Andy's next running goal is to complete a full marathon with his pal Seth.

information on your favorite charity—perhaps your personal tribute or dedication to a cancer survivor or a terminally ill child. The page can also list event information, race route, ideal locations to observe and cheer for you, funds raised to date, race goals, fund goals, total miles and special comments.

STAYING ACTIVE

Whether you choose to enter events or not, and whether you wish to continue running or not, completing the 13-week RunWalk program will have helped you increase your fitness level and gain new appreciation for the virtues and joys of exercise. There's always more to learn about fitness in general and running in particular, and you can continue to expand your knowledge by reading, attending conferences and events, signing up for seminars, joining a running group or just chatting with friends who have similar interests.

Whatever you decide to do, try and make exercise a part of your life. You'll be happier and healthier because of it, and in the end that's what makes it all worthwhile. To help you decide on your next steps, here are some scenarios you might find yourself in and possible programs to go with them. Find the option that's right for you.

1. **I completed the 13-week RunWalk program with success!** Fantastic! To solidify your newfound running fitness, do a month of maintenance running before you decide on your next challenge.

Week 1: DAY 1: 20 minutes
DAY 2: 40 minutes
DAY 3: 60 minutes

Week 2: DAY 1: 20 minutes
DAY 2: 30 minutes
DAY 3: 40 minutes

Repeat these sessions for at least two more weeks.

2. **I completed the 13-week RunWalk program but had some difficulty.**

   That happens to many people. Recommit to the 13-week Run-Walk program, but instead of going back to the beginning, start in Week 5. Allow yourself eight weeks to repeat and solidify that 10-k distance.

3. **I completed the program with a 10-k RunWalk event, and I'd like to experience another RunWalk event.**

   Congratulations! Source another event through an online running event calendar. You'll discover there are events everywhere in the world to consider! If you want some variety, consider 3 k, 5 k, 10 k and other odd distances or a trail-running or cross-country event. Whatever race you choose, consider supporting your favorite charitable cause.

4. **I'd like to run faster!**

   Great! Before you begin the 13-week RunFaster program (Appendix C), do a month of maintenance running to solidify your running fitness.

   Week 1: DAY 1: 20 minutes
   DAY 2: 40 minutes
   DAY 3: 60 minutes

   Week 2: DAY 1: 20 minutes
   DAY 2: 30 minutes
   DAY 3: 40 minutes

   Repeat these sessions for at least two more weeks.

5. **I'd like to run farther!**

   That's a common feeling. If you completed the 10-k distance comfortably, you're ready to embark on a half-marathon journey and can begin in Week 14 of the SportMedBC Half-Marathon program. Before you begin, chat with your family and friends so that you have their support. To complete the half-marathon training, you'll need twice as much time for workouts three times per week as you've been committing to the 13-week RunWalk program, and you may also feel more tired because of the increased exercise. Before you begin, check with your doctor to make sure you're healthy and have no underlying aches and pains that might be made worse by running farther.

6. **I'd like to complete a marathon now!**
   Wow, that's a wonderful idea if you've had no difficulty with this 13-week RunWalk program. We recommend that you stay conservative, though, and start with SportMedBC's Half-Marathon program. (See *Marathon and Half-Marathon: The Beginner's Guide.*) This will build your stamina gradually and allow your body to get used to the impact, keeping you injury free.

7. **I'm more comfortable walking than running.**
   Work through the 13-week program again, following the RunWalk option which progresses to 10 minutes of running broken up with a minute of walking. If you completed the running option last time around, you'll enjoy how easy the 10-k RunWalk option feels. Many people stay with "10-and-ones" forever and go on to complete marathons and other long-distance races using this repeated pattern.

8. **I'd like to continue running, but I can only commit to two days per week.**
   That's okay. You can maintain your running fitness on two days per week: go for 20 to 30 minutes one day and for 30 to 40 minutes the next. Consider adding another day of aerobic activity—swimming or pool running, cycling, brisk walking, cross-country skiing, using the elliptical trainer—to keep up your current level of fitness.

9. **I'd like to add some upper body work to my RunWalk fitness.**

That's a great idea. Add one or two days per week of a non-weight-bearing strength and conditioning activity, such as Pilates, yoga, tai chi or qigong.

10. **I'd like to add a dance class to my regular running program.**

Adding a weight-bearing (impact) strength and/or aerobic activity is always a good idea! You've achieved a base level of fitness that will allow you to try virtually any activity. The only limit is how you feel.

11. **I only want to run. I'm not interested in doing any other activity.**

That's okay. You are gaining strength and fitness through-out your body when you run but, in the long term, you risk developing overuse injuries and becoming bored if there is no variety in your activity. If that happens, you can choose to add other activities at that time.

12. **I'd like variety beyond running in my activity plan.**

You're not alone. Variety makes exercise interesting and encourages you to stick with it. Depending on how many days a week you like to exercise, here are a few options to optimize variety.

> three days/week: two days running, one day another aerobic activity
> four days/week: two days running, one day weight training, one day another aerobic activity
> five days/week: two days running, two days weight training, one day another aerobic activity
> six days/week: three days running, two days weight training, one day another aerobic activity

FACT

Of those surveyed, 68 percent of RunWalk participants go on to participate in other sports and activities.

13. I'd like to exercise every day.

Give yourself a break. The body needs at least one day off per week, though active rest such as walking the dog is okay on that day. In addition, it's important to build a holiday into your program: plan at least two weeks in the year when you don't exercise—or at least when you're active but not scheduled. When you start back, you'll feel newly motivated. A good way to do this might be to plan a "destination" race and spend a holiday there after the event. You'll feel like you've earned the right to kick back and relax.

A sample weekly program for the active person

MONDAY	45-minute run (on a trail in the park)
TUESDAY	25-minute swim (front crawl)
WEDNESDAY	50-minute run (steady pace)
THURSDAY	weight-training session (10 exercises, three sets each)
FRIDAY	45-minute run (varying pace)
SATURDAY	weight-training session (10 exercises, three sets each)
SUNDAY	Rest

CHAPTER 11 SUMMARY

1. You can easily maintain your 13-week RunWalk cardio fitness by exercising aerobically three times a week for 30 to 40 minutes.
2. Interval training, tempo running, hill and fartlek training are the four running workouts used to build strength and improve speed.
3. Participating in races can be a good way to stay motivated,

have fun, meet other runners, learn more about the sport and discover new places.

4. Charity runs can be a good way to stay fit and give back to the community at the same time.

5. The 13-week RunWalk program is only the beginning of your active lifestyle: continue to follow the program or modify it to suit your time, goals and interests.

Appendix A

STRETCHING EXERCISES

Here are some stretches for the major muscle groups used in running and walking. Use these stretches as a guide to building your own routine. It's a good idea to work systematically from the calves up to the shoulders (or vice versa).

Before stretching, always start with five to 10 minutes of jogging on the spot or slow and easy running to warm your muscles. Then move into your pre-training stretching exercises. Hold each position (no bouncing) for approximately 10 seconds. Your stretching routine should take no more than three to five minutes.

After your workout, use these same stretches to cool down. If you wish to work on increasing your flexibility, hold the stretches longer—anywhere from 15 seconds to three minutes—and repeat each stretch two to three times. Pay particular attention to the areas that you feel are the tightest; in runners these are usually the low back, hamstrings and calves.

Calf

1. Stand facing a wall, an arm's length plus 6 in (15 cm) away.
2. Place your right foot forward, halfway to the wall, and bend your right knee while keeping your left leg straight.
3. Lean into the wall, using your forearms for support and letting your left heel lift off the floor while keeping your head, neck, spine, pelvis and left leg in a straight line.
4. Exhale and shift your weight toward the wall while you attempt to press your left heel to the ground and your right knee toward the wall.
5. Hold the stretch and relax.
6. Repeat starting with your left leg forward.

Hamstring

This exercise requires a doorway.

1. Lie flat on your back, through a doorway, positioning your hips slightly in front of the door frame, with the inside of your lower right thigh against one side of the door frame.
2. Keeping your right leg straight and flat on the floor, exhale and raise your left leg up until your heel rests against the door frame. Do not bend your left knee.
3. Hold the stretch and relax.
4. To increase the stretch, slide your buttocks closer to the door frame, or lift the leg away from the door frame to create a right angle.
5. Repeat with your right leg raised.

Iliotibial Band

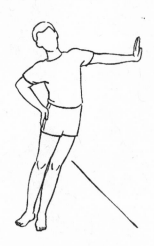

1. Stand with your left side toward a wall, an arm's length away, feet together.
2. Extend your left arm sideways at shoulder height so the flat of your hand is against the wall and you are leaning toward it.
3. Place your right hand on the side of your right hip.
4. Exhale, keeping your legs straight, tightening your buttocks and pushing your left hip in toward the wall until you feel the stretch down the outside of your left leg.
5. Hold the stretch and relax.
6. Repeat on the right side.

Quadriceps

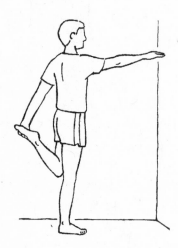

Avoid this exercise if it causes pain in your knee joint.

1. Stand facing a wall, an arm's length away. Place your right hand against the wall for balance and support.
2. Bend your left leg at the knee and raise the foot behind you until you can grasp it with your left hand.
3. Slightly bend your right leg at the knee and be sure to keep your lower back straight.
4. Pull your left heel toward your buttock.
5. Hold the stretch and relax.
6. Repeat with your right leg.

Groin

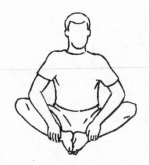

1. Sit upright on the floor, with your back against a wall.
2. Bend your knees up then let them fall to the sides with the soles of your feet facing each other.
3. Grasp your ankles with both hands and pull your heels toward your buttocks.
4. Rest your elbows on the inside of your thighs.
5. Slowly push your knees toward the floor until you feel the stretch in your groin.
6. Hold the stretch and relax.

Hip Flexor

(For those who are unable to kneel, this exercise can be done while sitting on the edge of a chair, and assuming the same position as illustrated but without the knee touching the ground.)

1. Stand with your feet together, then take one stride forward with your right foot.
2. Flexing your right knee, slowly lower your body toward the ground, finishing with your left knee touching the floor and your right heel flat on the floor.
3. Rest your hands just above the right knee and keep that knee bent at no more than a right angle.
4. For some, getting into this position will be enough. If you wish to increase the stretch, exhale while pushing your left hip forward and increasing the stretch on the left side.
5. Hold the stretch and relax.
6. Repeat with your left foot forward.

Gluteal

1. Lie flat on your back with your legs straight and arms out to the sides.
2. Bend the left knee and raise it toward your chest, grasping your leg under the knee or thigh with your right hand.
3. Keep your head, shoulders and elbows flat on the floor.
4. Exhale as you pull your knee across your body toward the floor.
5. Hold the stretch and relax.
6. Repeat with the right leg.

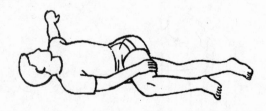

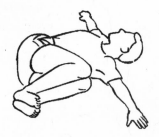

Lower Back

1. Lie flat on your back with your knees bent to form a right angle and your arms out to the sides.
2. Exhale and slowly lower both knees to the left side.
3. Keep your elbows, head and shoulders flat on the floor.
4. Hold the stretch and relax.
5. Repeat on the left side.

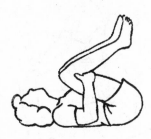

Lower Back

1. Lie flat on your back with your legs straight out.
2. Bend your knees and slide your heels toward your buttocks.
3. Using both hands, grasp behind your knees. (It's not important to keep your knees together—they should be comfortable.)
4. Exhale, pulling your knees toward your chest and slowly lifting your hips from the floor, while keeping your head and shoulders on the floor.
5. Hold the stretch and relax.

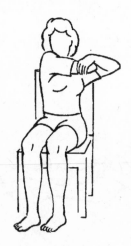

Shoulder

1. Sit with your right arm raised in front of you at shoulder height.
2. Bring your right hand across your chest and place it on the back of your left shoulder, keeping your elbow at shoulder height.
3. Grasp your right elbow with your left hand.
4. Exhale and pull your elbow in toward your left shoulder.
5. Hold the stretch and relax.
6. Repeat with your left arm.

STRENGTH-TRAINING EXERCISES

Strength training is beneficial for runners of all ages—at any level of performance. Here are some sample exercises for starting a strength-training program.

Before starting a new routine, consult a fitness professional experienced in designing these programs. Aim for two or three strength-training sessions per week.

Start your workout with a proper warm-up: some low-intensity aerobic activity such as stationary cycling, walking or light jogging, followed by some light stretching. Then, begin holding lighter weights during these lower-body exercises. How light? Consult a professional to find out what's right for you. If you don't have anyone to ask, make sure you can lift the weight with little effort for at least 10 repetitions. Err on the side of caution.

As a general guideline, start by doing one or two sets of 10 to 15 repetitions for each exercise—do the minimum number of repetitions in the beginning and build your way up to the maximum. As you become more confident and competent, gradually increase the weight or resistance.

LOWER BODY

Lunges

1. Stand tall with your hands on your hips and your feet shoulder-width apart.
2. Keep your back straight and your head up.
3. Step forward slowly with your left leg. Bend your left knee and lower your body forward and down so that your weight is over this knee. Make sure that your kneecap does not extend past your toes. Keep your back leg relaxed and slightly bent so that your knee almost touches the floor. Your trunk should remain upright. Step backward to the start position.
4. Exhale as you step forward and inhale as you return to the start position.
5. Repeat this exercise with your right leg.

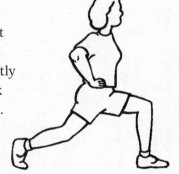

Step-Ups

1. Stand tall with your feet shoulder-width apart.
2. Keep your back straight (flat) and your head upright, eyes looking forward.
3. Step up with your right leg on a bench, box or other stable platform.
4. The height of the platform will depend on your strength and level of fitness. The maximum height of your platform should not exceed the level required to place your femur (thigh bone) in a horizontal position.
5. Once your right foot is firmly on the platform, shift your hips forward and step up on the platform using only your right leg, until you are in a fully erect posture.
6. Follow through with the trailing leg.
7. Step down, first with the right leg, then with the left leg.
8. Repeat the sequence 10 times with a right-leg lead and follow 10 times with a left-leg lead.
9. Remember to exhale as you step up and inhale as you step down.

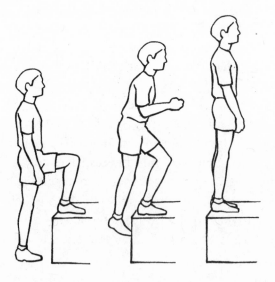

Squats

1. Stand tall with your feet shoulder-width apart.
2. Keeping your back flat, move your hips back and down slowly until your thigh bone (femur) is horizontal.
3. In the squat position, your knees should not line up ahead of your toes, and your head should be in a neutral position with your eyes looking forward.
4. Slowly return to a standing position and then repeat the sequence.
5. Exhale as you ascend and inhale as you descend.

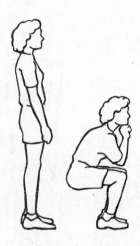

ABDOMINALS

Abdominal Crunches

1. Lie face up on the floor with your lower legs resting on an exercise ball (or a chair).
2. Position your body so that your thighs are at a 90-degree angle.
3. Folding your arms across your chest, curl your body toward your thighs until your upper back is off the floor. Slowly return to the start position. Be careful not to bounce or jerk your body.
4. Exhale as you curl up, and inhale as you return to the start position.

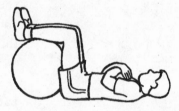

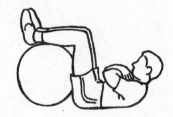

UPPER BODY

Shoulder Press

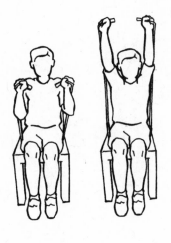

1. Sit tall in a chair with your feet in front of your knees. Be sure that your back does not touch the back of the chair.
2. Keep your back straight and your head up.
3. Sit on the middle of the band and hold one end of the elastic in each hand.
4. Push both hands overhead simultaneously to a fully extended position.
5. Return your hands to shoulder height, making a V-position with the band.
6. Your hands should maintain a palms-forward position throughout the movement.
7. Repeat this sequence 10 times.
8. Exhale through the push phase and inhale as you return your hands to the shoulder position.
9. You can adjust the resistance by lengthening or shortening the elastic.

Lat Pulldown

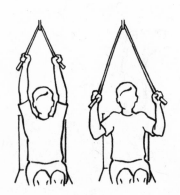

1. Sit tall in a chair with your feet in front of your knees and your back not touching the back of the chair.
2. Keep your back straight with your head up and eyes forward.
3. Hold the ends of the elastic, one in each hand with the middle of the band looped over an overhead object (e.g., a coat hook).
4. In a start position with the arms extended and hands overhead, palms facing forward, pull downward until your hands reach a shoulder position.
5. Release slowly, allowing the elastic to pull your hands back into an overhead position.
6. Repeat this sequence 10 times.
7. Exhale through the push phase and inhale as you return your hands to the shoulder position.
8. You can adjust the resistance by lengthening or shortening the elastic.

Chest Press

1. Sit tall in a chair with your feet in front of your knees and your back not touching the back of the chair.
2. Keep your back straight, your head up and eyes forward.
3. Hold the ends of the elastic, one in each hand, with the middle of the band looped behind your back.
4. With your hands at chest level in a palms-forward position, press forward (horizontally) to an arms-fully-extended position.
5. Release slowly, allowing the elastic to return your hands to the chest level.
6. Repeat this sequence 10 times.
7. Exhale through the push phase and inhale as you return your hands to the shoulder position.
8. You can adjust the resistance by lengthening or shortening the elastic.

Seated Row

1. Sit tall in a chair with your feet in front of your knees and your back not touching the back of the chair.
2. Keep your back straight, your head up and your eyes forward.
3. Hold the ends of the elastic, one in each hand, with the middle of the band looped around an object directly in front of you (e.g., a doorknob, table leg).
4. Begin with your arms extended horizontally and palms facing the floor.
5. Pull your hands back to a mid-chest position.
6. Release slowly, allowing the elastic to return your arms to a fully extended and horizontal position.
7. Repeat this sequence 10 times.
8. Exhale through the push phase and inhale as you return your hands to the shoulder position.
9. You can adjust the resistance by lengthening or shortening the elastic.

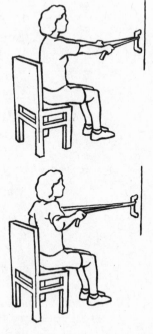

Appendix B

....

THE 13-WEEK RUNWALK MAINTENANCE PROGRAM

This program is designed for people who have completed the 13-week RunWalk program and want to maintain their fitness gains by staying active. You may choose to follow this program, a modified version of this program or another program altogether. Whichever you choose, remember that if you have a specific training program to follow you will be more likely to maintain your activity level.

As with the other programs in this book, you will have three training sessions each week. It's best to schedule these throughout the week so that you have at least one day between sessions. Most training sessions will take about an hour to complete.

Note that the times shown do not include your five-minute warm-up and five-minute cool-down in each training session. Be sure to allow extra time in your schedule for these essential components of your training.

WEEK 1

☐ **Session 1** (42 minutes)
Run four minutes. Walk two minutes. Do this seven times.

☐ **Session 2** (48 minutes)
Run four minutes. Walk two minutes. Do this eight times.

☐ **Session 3** (48 minutes)
Run four minutes. Walk two minutes. Do this eight times.

WEEK 2

☐ **Session 1** (42 minutes)
Walk five minutes. Walk one minute. Do this seven times.

☐ **Session 2** (48 minutes)
Run five minutes. Walk one minute. Do this eight times.

☐ **Session 3** (54 minutes)
Run five minutes. Walk one minute. Do this nine times.

WEEK 3

☐ **Session 1** (45 minutes)
Run seven minutes. Walk two minutes. Do this five times.

☐ **Session 2** (45 minutes)
Run seven minutes. Walk two minutes. Do this five times.

☐ **Session 3** (54 minutes)
Run seven minutes. Walk two minutes. Do this six times.

WEEK 4

☐ **Session 1** (44 minutes)
Run 10 minutes. Walk one minute. Do this four times.

☐ **Session 2** (52 minutes)
Run 12 minutes. Walk one minute. Do this four times.

☐ **Session 3** (44 minutes)
Run 10 minutes. Walk one minute. Do this four times.

WEEK 5

☐ **Session 1** (48 minutes)
Run 15 minutes. Walk one minute. Do this three times.

☐ **Session 2** (51 minutes)
Run 16 minutes. Walk one minute. Do this three times.

☐ **Session 3** (54 minutes)
Run 17 minutes. Walk one minute. Do this three times.

WEEK 6

☐ **Session 1** (41 minutes)
Run 20 minutes. Walk one minute. Run 20 minutes.

☐ **Session 2** (43 minutes)
Run 22 minutes. Walk one minute. Run 20 minutes.

☐ **Session 3** (43 minutes)
Run 22 minutes. Walk one minute. Run 20 minutes.

☐ **Session 1** (30 minutes)
Run 30 minutes.

☐ **Session 2** (30 minutes)
Run 30 minutes.

☐ **Session 3** (35 minutes)
Run 35 minutes.

WEEK 8

☐ **Session 1** (33 minutes)
Run 33 minutes.

☐ **Session 2** (30 minutes)
Run 30 minutes.

☐ **Session 3** (35 minutes)
Run 35 minutes.

WEEK 9

☐ **Session 1** (41 minutes)
Run 30 minutes. Walk one minute. Run 10 minutes.

☐ **Session 2** (46 minutes)
Run 30 minutes. Walk one minute. Run 15 minutes.

☐ **Session 3** (46 minutes)
Run 30 minutes. Walk one minute. Run 15 minutes.

WEEK 10

☐ **Session 1** (46 minutes)
Run 35 minutes. Walk one minute. Run 10 minutes.

☐ **Session 2** (51 minutes)
Run 30 minutes. Walk one minute. Run 20 minutes.

☐ **Session 3** (51 minutes)
Run 30 minutes. Walk one minute. Run 20 minutes.

WEEK 11

☐ **Session 1** (40 minutes)
Run 40 minutes.

☐ **Session 2** (45 minutes)
Run 45 minutes.

☐ **Session 3** (40 minutes)
Run 40 minutes.

WEEK 12

☐ **Session 1** (56 minutes)
Run 45 minutes. Walk one minute. Run 10 minutes.

☐ **Session 2** (61 minutes)
Run 45 minutes. Walk one minute. Run 15 minutes.

☐ **Session 3** (40 minutes)
Run 24 minutes. Walk one minute. Run 15 minutes.

☐ **Session 1** (35 minutes)
Run 35 minutes.

☐ **Session 2** (40 minutes)
Run 40 minutes.

☐ **Session 3** (60 minutes)
Complete a 10-k event (if this is your goal) or run 60 minutes.

Appendix C

....

THE 13-WEEK RUN FASTER PROGRAM

This program is designed for people who have completed the 13-week RunWalk program and would like to increase their running endurance and intensity in a safe and effective way. Anyone following this program should be sure to allow at least one rest (or cross training) day in between any two running sessions.

Note: be sure to complete your prescribed warm-up and cooldown in each training session. These are essential components of your training.

WEEK 1

☐ **Session 1** (44 minutes)

WARM-UP: Jog slowly 10 minutes.

Run briskly three minutes. Jog slowly two minutes.

Run briskly two minutes. Jog slowly two minutes.

Run briskly one minute. Jog slowly two minutes.

Do this two times.

COOL-DOWN: Jog slowly 10 minutes.

☐ **Session 2** (30 minutes).

WARM-UP: Jog slowly five minutes.

Run 20 minutes.

COOL-DOWN: Jog slowly five minutes.

☐ **Session 3** (35 minutes)

WARM-UP: Jog slowly five minutes.

Run 25 minutes.

COOL-DOWN: Jog slowly five minutes.

WEEK 2

☐ **Session 1** (44 minutes)

WARM-UP: Jog slowly 10 minutes.

Run briskly two minutes. Jog slowly two minutes.

Do this six times.

COOL-DOWN: Jog slowly 10 minutes.

☐ **Session 2** (30 minutes)

WARM-UP: Jog slowly five minutes.

Run 20 minutes.

COOL-DOWN: Jog slowly five minutes.

☐ **Session 3** (40 minutes)

WARM-UP: Jog slowly five minutes.

Run 30 minutes.

COOL-DOWN: Jog slowly five minutes.

NOTE

Brisk running means you should not be able to speak any more than two sentences at a time. Any more and you're going too slow; any less and you're going too fast.

WEEK 3

☐ **Session 1** (50 minutes)
WARM-UP: Jog slowly 10 minutes.
Run briskly one minute. Jog slowly two minutes.
Do this 10 times.
COOL-DOWN: Jog slowly 10 minutes.

☐ **Session 2** (30 minutes)
WARM-UP: Jog slowly five minutes.
Run 20 minutes.
COOL-DOWN: Jog slowly five minutes.

☐ **Session 3** (45 minutes)
WARM-UP: Jog slowly five minutes.
Run 35 minutes.
COOL-DOWN: Jog slowly five minutes.

WEEK 4 (Recovery Week)

☐ **Session 1** (45 minutes)
WARM-UP: Jog slowly 10 minutes.
Run 25 minutes.
COOL-DOWN: Jog slowly 10 minutes.

☐ **Session 2** (30 minutes)
WARM-UP: Jog slowly five minutes.
Run 20 minutes.
COOL-DOWN: Jog slowly five minutes.

☐ **Session 3** (40 minutes)
WARM-UP: Jog slowly five minutes.
Run 30 minutes.
COOL-DOWN: Jog slowly five minutes.

WEEK 5

☐ **Session 1** (55 minutes)
WARM-UP: Jog slowly 10 minutes.
Run briskly five minutes. Jog slowly two minutes.
Do this five times.
COOL-DOWN: Jog slowly 10 minutes.

☐ **Session 2** (30 minutes)
WARM-UP: Jog slowly five minutes.
Run 20 minutes.
COOL-DOWN: Jog slowly five minutes.

☐ **Session 3** (40–50 minutes)
WARM-UP: Jog slowly five minutes.
Run 30–40 minutes.
COOL-DOWN: Jog slowly five minutes.

You are now beginning to know yourself better as a runner. To support that independence, in Sessions 2 and 3 you will now have the option to vary your distance slightly, depending on how you feel. Enjoy some freedom, but stay within the suggested time parameter and choose the shorter options if you are a beginner.

WEEK 6

☐ **Session 1** (60 minutes)
WARM-UP: Jog slowly 10 minutes.
Run 40-minute change-of-pace fartlek.
COOL-DOWN: Jog slowly 10 minutes.

☐ **Session 2** (30–40 minutes)
WARM-UP: Jog slowly five minutes.
Run 20–30 minutes.
COOL-DOWN: Jog slowly five minutes.

☐ **Session 3** (40–50 minutes)
WARM-UP: Jog slowly five minutes.
Run 30–40 minutes.
COOL-DOWN: Jog slowly five minutes.

Fartlek is the Swedish word for "speed play." Have fun with this workout. Try different speeds and distances in intervals. Anything goes: short intervals of a minute or less, or longer intervals as you feel stronger. Recover by jogging slowly between intervals. You could even do exercises like sit-ups and push-ups!

WEEK 7

☐ **Session 1** (about 50 minutes or 5-k distance at 10-k pace)
WARM-UP: Jog slowly 10 minutes.
Run 30 minutes or 5 k.
COOL-DOWN: Jog slowly 10 minutes.

☐ **Session 2** (30–40 minutes)
WARM-UP: Jog slowly five minutes.
Run 20–30 minutes.
COOL-DOWN: Jog slowly five minutes.

☐ **Session 3** (50–60 minutes)
WARM-UP: Jog slowly five minutes.
Run 40–50 minutes.
COOL-DOWN: Jog slowly five minutes.

WEEK 8 (Recovery Week)

☐ **Session 1** (60 minutes)
WARM-UP: Jog slowly 10 minutes.
Run 40 minutes.
COOL-DOWN: Jog slowly 10 minutes.

☐ **Session 2** (30 minutes)
WARM-UP: Jog slowly five minutes.
Run 20 minutes.
COOL-DOWN: Jog slowly five minutes.

☐ **Session 3** (40 minutes)
WARM-UP: Jog slowly five minutes.
Run 30 minutes.
COOL-DOWN: Jog slowly five minutes.

WEEK 9

☐ **Session 1** (74 minutes)
WARM-UP: Jog slowly 10 minutes.
Run briskly five minutes. Jog slowly five minutes.
Run briskly three minutes. Jog slowly two minutes.
Run briskly one minute. Jog slowly two minutes.
Do this three times.
COOL-DOWN: Jog slowly 10 minutes.

☐ **Session 2** (30–40 minutes)
WARM-UP: Jog slowly five minutes.
Run 20–30 minutes.
COOL-DOWN: Jog slowly five minutes.

☐ **Session 3** (50–60 minutes)
WARM-UP: Jog slowly five minutes.
Run 40–50 minutes.
COOL-DOWN: Jog slowly five minutes.

WEEK 10

☐ **Session 1** (70 minutes)
WARM-UP: Jog slowly 10 minutes.
Run briskly three minutes. Jog slowly two minutes.
Do this 10 times.
COOL-DOWN: Jog slowly 10 minutes.

☐ **Session 2** (30–40 minutes)
WARM-UP: Jog slowly five minutes.
Run 20–30 minutes.
COOL-DOWN: Jog slowly five minutes.

☐ **Session 3** (50–60 minutes)
WARM-UP: Jog slowly five minutes.
Run 40–50 minutes.
COOL-DOWN: Jog slowly five minutes.

WEEK 11

☐ **Session 1** (64–76 minutes)

WARM-UP: Jog slowly 10 minutes.

Hill option: On a 25-degree slope, run briskly uphill one minute. Jog slowly back downhill. Do this eight times. On the same hill, run briskly uphill 30 seconds. Jog slowly back downhill. Do this eight times.

No-hill option: Run briskly two minutes. Jog slowly two minutes. Do this eight times.

Run briskly one minute. Jog slowly two minutes. Do this eight times.

COOL-DOWN: Jog slowly 10 minutes.

☐ **Session 2** (40–50 minutes)

WARM-UP: Jog slowly five minutes.

Run 30–40 minutes.

COOL-DOWN: Jog slowly five minutes.

☐ **Session 3** (60–70 minutes)

WARM-UP: Jog slowly five minutes.

Run 50–60 minutes.

COOL-DOWN: Jog slowly five minutes.

WEEK 12

☐ **Session 1** (60 minutes)
WARM-UP: Jog slowly 10 minutes.
Run 40 minutes.
COOL-DOWN: Jog slowly 10 minutes.

☐ **Session 2** (30–40 minutes)
WARM-UP: Jog slowly five minutes.
Run 20–30 minutes.
COOL-DOWN: Jog slowly five minutes.

☐ **Session 3** (40–50 minutes)
WARM-UP: Jog slowly five minutes.
Run 30–40 minutes.
COOL-DOWN: Jog slowly five minutes.

WEEK 13 (This is it!)

☐ **Session 1** (44 minutes)
WARM-UP: Jog slowly 10 minutes.
Run briskly three minutes. Jog slowly two minutes.
Run briskly two minutes. Jog slowly two minutes.
Run briskly one minute. Jog slowly two minutes.
Do this two times.
COOL-DOWN: Jog slowly 10 minutes.

☐ **Session 2** (30 minutes)
WARM-UP: Jog slowly five minutes.
Run 20 minutes.
COOL-DOWN: Jog slowly five minutes.

☐ **Session 3** (Event Day 10-k)
Run as you feel.
Have fun and take care not to start too quickly.
Congratulations!

Resources
and References

·····································

Health, Exercise and Physiology
Books

Tucker, R., and J. Dugas. *The Runner's Body: How the Latest Sport Science Can Help You Run Stronger, Longer and Faster.* Emmaus, PA: Rodale, 2009.

Bushman, Barbara, and American College of Sports Medicine. *ACSM's Complete Guide to Fitness and Health.* Champaign, IL: Human Kinetics, 2011.

Wilmore, J., and D. Costill. *Physiology of Sport and Exercise.* Champaign, IL: Human Kinetics, 2007.

Referenced Articles in Journals

Chave, S.P.W., J.N. Morris, S. Moss and A.M. Semmence. "Vigorous Exercise in Leisure Time and the Death Rate: A Study of Male Civil Servants." *Journal of Epidemiology and Community Health* 32 (1978): 239–43.

Paffenbarger, R.S., R.T. Hyde, D.L. Jung and A.L. Wing. "Epidemiology of Exercise and Coronary Heart Disease." *Clinics in Sports Medicine* 3 no. 2 (1984): 297–318.

Injury Prevention and Treatment
Books

Noakes, T., and S. Granger. *Running Injuries: How to Prevent Them & Overcome Them.* Cape Town: Oxford University Press, 2003.

Dreyer, Danny, and K. Dreyer. *ChiRunning: A Revolutionary Approach to Effortless, Injury-Free Running.* New York: Fireside, 2009.

Maharam, Lewis. *Running Doc's Guide to Healthy Running: How to Fix Injuries, Stay Active and Run Pain-Free*. Boulder, CO: Velo Press, 2011.

Referenced Articles in Journals

Kerrigan et al. "The Effect of Running Shoes on Lower Extremity Joint." *American Academy of Physical Medicine and Rehabilitation* 1, December 2009, 1058–63.

Macintyre, J., and D.R. Lloyd-Smith. "Intrinsic Factors in Overuse Running Injuries." In *Sports Injuries: Basic Principles of Prevention and Care*, edited by Per Renstrom. International Olympic Committee Encyclopedia Series no. 4. Oxford: Blackwell Scientific Publications, 1993: 139–60.

Motivation and Psychology

Mahoney, Kirk. *Mental Tricks for Endurance Runners and Walkers*. Charleston, SC: CreateSpace, 2010.

Orlick, Terry. *In Pursuit of Excellence, 4th Edition*. Champaign, IL: Human Kinetics, 2007.

SportMedBC. *RunWalk Training Logbook*. www.sportmedbc.com, 2011.

Nutrition

Chuey, Patricia, E. Campbell and M. Waisman. *Simply Great Food: 250 Quick, Easy and Delicious Recipes*. Toronto: Robert Rose, 2009.

Clark, Nancy. *Nancy Clark's Sports Nutrition Guidebook*. Champaign, IL: Human Kinetics, 2008.

Clark, Nancy. *Nancy Clark's Food Guide for New Runners: Getting it Right from the Start*. Aachen, Germany: Meyer & Meyer Fachverlag und Buchhandel GmbH, 2009.

Waisman, M. *Dietitians of Canada Cook!* Toronto: Robert Rose, 2011.

Running (General)

Bingham, John. *The Courage to Start: A Guide to Running for Your Life*. New York: Simon & Schuster, 1999.

Caron, Marnie, and The Sport Medicine Council of British Columbia. *Marathon and Half-Marathon: The Beginner's Guide*. Vancouver: Greystone Books, 2006.

Caron, Marnie, and the Sport Medicine Council of British Columbia. *Walking for Fitness: The Beginner's Handbook*. Vancouver: Greystone Books, 2007.

Douglas, Scott. *The Little Red Book of Running*. New York: Skyhorse Publishing, 2011.

McDougall, Christopher. *Born to Run: A Hidden Tribe, Superathletes, and the Greatest Race the World Has Never Seen*. New York: Random House, 2009.

Stanton, John. *Running*. Toronto: Penguin Canada, 2011.

Running the World Series (Blaze Travel Guides ebooks—various).

Strength and Conditioning

Alter, Michael J. *The Science of Flexibility,* 3rd ed. Champaign, IL: Human Kinetics, 2004.

Musnick, D., and M. Pierce. *Conditioning for Outdoor Fitness: Functional Fitness and Nutrition for Every Body.* Seattle: The Mountaineers Books, 2004.

Women's Health

Nordahl, K. *Fit to Deliver.* www.fittodeliver.com, 2000.

Physiotherapy Association of British Columbia. *Your Body After Baby: Things to Consider After Having Your Baby.* http://classic.bcphysio.org/pdfs/Postpartumflyer.pdf

Online

Websites

American Dietetic Association
www.eatright.org
Gatorade Sport Science Institute
www.gssiweb.com
The Vegetarian Resource Group
www.vrg.org
Nancy Clark, Sports Nutritionist
www.nancyclarkrd.com
United States Department of Agriculture, Food and Nutrition Information Center
www.nal.usda.gov/fnic
Runner's World
www.runnersworld.com
Runner's World for Women
www.womens-running.com
SportMedBC
www.sportmedbc.com

Online Running Communities

SportMedBC www.sportmedbc.com
Access our logbooks and the latest training resources for runners and walkers.
Runners' Lounge www.runnerslounge.com
Map my Run www.mapmyrun.com
Tribal Running www.tribalrunning.net

Runner's World www.runnersworld.com
Running Room www.runningroom.com
Nike http://nikerunning.nike.com
New Balance http://www.newbalance.com/live/

Running Apps
RunKeeper (free)
Using your phone's GPS, track your fitness activities, including distance, time, pace, calories, heart rate and path traveled on a map.
RunningMap Trackometer, $1.99
Track and share running routes with your friends, and add photos and mark points of interest.

Index

heart rate, 11, 12, 13, 60, 71,
157, 163
heat and injuries, 138
heel pain, 142
hill running/training, 101–3, 166,
167–68
hitting the wall, 17
hot-weather running, 40–41
hypoglycemia (low blood
sugar), 125

I

icing injuries, 138
iliotibial band syndrome, 141, 184
illness and exercise, 30, 61, 151
immune system, 10, 14, 18
injuries. *see also* pain: coming back
after, 146–47; elastic tension
bandages, 139; RICE treatment,
137–39; stress fractures, 17, 119,
145; swelling of, 137; types of,
139–46
in-line skating, 97–98
interval training, 162, 166, 169–70
iron, dietary, 75, 112, 121–22, 122
"ironman" competitions, 174

J

jogging strollers, 82–85

K

Kanuka, Lynn, 4, 96, 149, 172
Kegels, 82
Kerrigan, Casey, 21
ketosis, 110
knee pain, 133–35, 140–41

L

lactic acid, 9, 81
Lee, Diane, 81
log, training, 32–33
low-carbohydrate diets, 109–11

M

Macintyre, Jim, 133–34, 135,
141, 145
MacLean, Dr. Christopher, 20,
21, 23
*Marathon and Half-Marathon: The
Beginner's Guide* (SportMedBC),
172, 173
marathons, full, 172, 174
marathons, half, 172, 173, 177–78
McDougall, Christopher, 21
medical conditions and exercise,
149–50, 155
merino wool clothing, 27
minerals, 112, 113, 114, 118–23,
120, 122
minimalist shoes, 23–24
moderation in training, 16,
94, 165
moderation with foods, 108, 130
Moore, Phil, 21, 27, 78
Morbey, Denise, 76, 79, 80,
82, 84
Morris, J.N., 6
motivation: barriers, 71, 162; goal
setting and, 29; maintaining, 162, 163, 166, 167, 169, 174;
train your mind, 61–71; warm-
ups, 69–70
muscle(s): abdominal, 81, 99, 189;
aging and muscle mass, 99;
balance, 94; soreness, 17, 36,
145–46; strength, 99, 102, 129;
tone, 12, 74, 99
muscles, core. *see* core exercises;
core strength

N

natural foods, 109, 124
Noakes, Dr. Tim, 16, 70, 91, 139,
140, 141
Nordahl, Dr. Karen, 74, 79, 80, 82

Check out these other health & fitness books

from GREYSTONE BOOKS and

the Sport Medicine Council of British Columbia

to get you on your way:

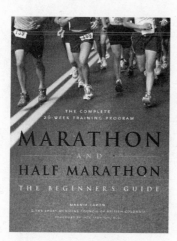

Marathon and Half Marathon

Building on the success of the popular *Beginning Runner's Handbook,* this practical, easy-to-use guide provides a step-by-step program for running the half or the full marathon for the first time.

PAPERBACK EDITION: 978-1-55365-158-1

EBOOK EDITION: 978-1-92668-529-8

$19.95

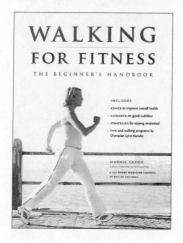

Walking for Fitness

Walk your way to good health with this comprehensive guide.

PAPERBACK EDITION: 978-1-55365-219-9

EBOOK EDITION: 978-1-92668-555-7

$19.95

Available everywhere books are sold.

each stretch 10 sec. 2-3 times / per muscle group